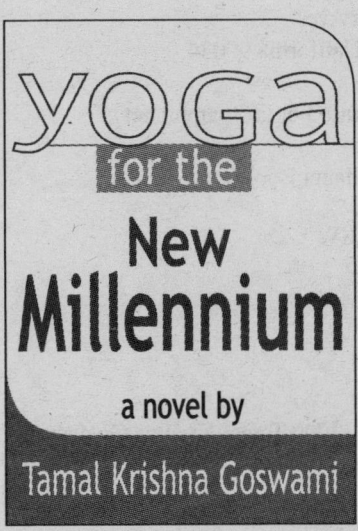

yoga for the New Millennium

a novel by

Tamal Krishna Goswami

THE BHAKTIVEDANTA BOOK TRUST

Los Angeles. London. Paris. Bombay. Sydney. Hong Kong

Readers interested in the subject matter of this book are invited by the publisher to corespond with its secretary at either of the following addresses:

The Bhaktivedanta Book Trust
3764 Watseka Ave.
Los angeles, California 90034
USA
    email info.bbt.la@pamho.net

The Bhaktivedanta Book Trust
P.O. Box 380,
Riverstone, NSW
Australia 2765

© 1989, 1994, 2000 Tamal Krishna Goswami
All Rights Reserved

Library of Congress Catalog Card Number: 94-96591

ISBN 0-9643485-0-0

Printed in Australia

Dedicated to
the people of China,
with the blessings of
His Divine Grace
A.C. Bhaktivedanta Swami Prabhupada,
my spiritual master

1

KUANG SHI WALKED BRISKLY, his stout legs proudly beating the pavement, his face flushed with excitement. He was happy to be on his way to see his Uncle Lawrence and Aunt Shiao Lin, although he wished he were in Beijing to share the news of his academic achievement with his old school friends. This cool and breezy April evening in New York City in fact reminded him of Beijing. The southern winds would have just begun to chase away the memories of winter, though the friendly winds could be equally ominous. The sky would fill with fine particles of earth from the surrounding plains, shrouding the entire city with a reddish-grey veil of powdered dust. But the dust clouds would soon clear to reveal a city festively decorated with pinkish-white cherry blossoms flowering in the daytime warmth. Spring was a season for celebration, and Kuang Shi was certainly in a mood to celebrate.

He was suddenly yanked back to New York City when he found himself about to walk smack into the front fender of a furiously honking Yellow Cab in the middle of the crosswalk at Fifty-ninth Street and Columbus Circle, which marked the southwest boundary of Central Park. Thinking of China always left him feeling slightly alienated, and the contrast between the two countries always overwhelmed him.

During summer vacations Kuang Shi had traveled throughout the United States, but nowhere had he found people so vibrant, cosmopolitan, and open-minded as they were here in New York. It was a melting pot, to be sure, fusing European, Latin, Asian, and African cultures together into an incredibly versatile population. Such diverse nationalities surcharged the cultural climate of the city. Here was a striking difference indeed between America and China: Only very recently had his countrymen even begun to mingle with foreigners. In the past they viewed foreign ways with scorn, proud of their own unquestioned superiority.

New York was the American city where most immigrants got their start: Chinatown, Little Italy, Harlem, and all the other ethnic areas. In the streets of New York it was not at all uncommon to hear Chinese, Italian, Russian, Spanish, Yiddish, or German intermingled with English. It simply depended on which part of the city you happened to find yourself in. But the children of the immigrants didn't always care to identify with their parents' origins and often laughed at the remnants of the traditions which they were trying to grow out of. Although their parents were not always pleased, they were nevertheless proud that their children were becoming real Americans. This was one of the main reasons that they had come to America—to build a future for their children, far better than what lay in store for them had they remained in their native lands.

From his first days in America he made special efforts to become Americanized; yet, it was painful for him to give up his Chinese ways. To help him alleviate this sense of separation from his homeland, he had deliberately sought out other Chinese students and often went with them to eat and breathe the atmosphere of Chinatown. Speaking in his native language gave him some solace and made him feel that he was not wholly disconnected from home. After all, Chinese traditions and values were ancient and venerable, having remained relatively unchanged through centuries while entire civilizations elsewhere had come and gone. Only after Liberation, during the past forty years or so, had there been any indication that the previously invulnerable traditions were actually subject to change; and of late, everyone, government man and peasant alike, was beginning to recognize that the principle of modernization and reform was not only inevitable, but desirable. Although his country might debate the effects of Western influence and the man in the street might speculate on what it was like to live in the West, Kuang Shi, before he left in 1983, had already concluded that China would never again be the same. The ancient past was now inextricably bound to the modern world. Five years in America had molded him into a byproduct of two vastly different cultures. Kuang Shi wondered if it had been a successful mutation.

It was not always so. During the first year everything seemed so strange; he constantly thought of returning home. But the ignominy of such an act was as obvious as were the advantages of remaining in America. His Chinese friends advised him to be patient: It takes time to adjust, they said. But it was his few close American friends at Columbia University, like Winston, David, Ann, and Red, who actually convinced him to stay on. A metamorphosis was unmistakable. A transformation was slowly occurring: Li Kuang Shi to Charlie Li, and soon Dr. Charles Li. His clothes, his manners, his fluent English with its characteristic American accent—these were the proof.

These changes in his life were not just internal, for now he was beginning to think very seriously of a permanent career in America. Just a week ago he had received a lucrative offer from Abbott Laboratories, the large pharmaceutical company based in Chicago. Following the one from Hoffmann-La Roche, it was the second such offer. After reviewing his Ph.D. dissertation abstract and the letters of recommendation from his instructors, as well as conducting extensive interviews with him in person, both companies were convinced he could make important contributions as the burgeoning field of genetic engineering prepared for the new millennium. A starting salary of one hundred thousand dollars! Hardly a soul in all of China could ever hope to earn so much. Research chemists like himself were lucky to get two hundred *yuan* a month! Moreover, it had struck him that since he had received a private rather than a government scholarship, he could convince himself that he was under no obligation to return home. After all, he had not taken any money from the Chinese government. He had received a full fellowship grant of more than twenty thousand dollars per year from the K. C. Wang Foundation of Hong Kong to attend one of the finest schools in America, Columbia University. And happily, the only condition was that the scholarship be repaid if he decided not to return to China. That didn't bother him. He would make more than enough in two years to pay everyone back!

Kuang Shi felt free to do as he liked: He was bound neither by legal nor financial restraints. The only hurdle was his father. He knew how patriotic his father could be, and he did not rule out the possibility of some officials in his native Guondoung province exerting some social pressure on his parents, which could very easily make his father lose face for having an unpatriotic son. Kuang Shi had no desire to disobey or even to be disloyal. He had simply been waiting for the right opportunity to write his parents. Now that his Ph.D. was imminent, he wanted to write them soon. He would try to convince them that staying in America allowed him to serve all humanity because of the preeminent status of American science.

Relations between the United States and China were improving so rapidly that thousands of Chinese students were now studying in universities all over the country. Schools competed strongly for the best of China's students, and nine out often of them would not be returning to China. It was a serious problem for his country. A real brain drain, he thought. But what else could they expect? Why should he return? He would never be able to realize his potential if he returned there. The chances of his getting a decent position were slim, for these were always awarded to those with seniority, even though they were often less qualified. He felt certain that there would be less encouragement for him to do the research that he was interested in, and even if there were, where would be the necessary facilities? His income would be so meager that he would probably have to take on a second job. He could make more money driving a taxi in Beijing than as a Ph.D. in biochemistry. He had made up his mind: He was not going back.

2

KUANG SHI SAW the horse-drawn carriages awaiting tourists along Central Park South. He was moving quickly toward the subway entrance at Fifty-ninth Street to take the IND line to Queens. He hadn't phoned his uncle Lawrence because he had wanted to surprise him personally with the news that his thesis had been accepted. As he crossed Columbus Circle, he saw something he had never seen before, a row of colorful tents made of blue and red-striped canvas, open at the front. As he neared them, Kuang Shi paused before a large banner that read "Festival of India." Was this another one of those cultural exchanges that the city was famous for?

The dozen or so tents seemed an unusual contrast to the grand and stately buildings towering in the background, lining Central Park. Whoever picked the spot couldn't have done better—right at the subway entrance! Hundreds of people were moving from one tent to another looking over the different exhibits.

Kuang Shi was in a hurry, but he had a few minutes to spare. He looked at some of what were mostly photographic displays, but one in particular caught his attention: "Changing Bodies"? It just didn't ring a bell, a series of life-size mannequins, painted and dressed so expertly they were lifelike, depicting a man at different stages of his life. The first was a small baby, the next an infant, the third a child. Hmmm... Changing bodies, interesting notion.

Kuang Shi took a few steps back and looked at the twenty or twenty-five figures, each marking a change of perhaps three or four years in a man's life. He looked for the one that was closest to his own age. It happened to be the one right in the middle, a man in the prime of life, strong, handsome, youthful. Kuang Shi noted he was holding some books—a student, no doubt. The look of worry written upon the very next figure's face was obvious. Perhaps he had married, Kuang Shi laughed to himself. Probably the added responsibilities of life, judging by his knit brow. By the next figure decline was setting in, the man's once upright posture now slumping slightly, his left hand raised upward as if holding off old age. Fear? Of what, Kuang Shi wondered. The answer came in the following figures, showing the man progressively growing older and older, his hair greying, then falling out, his body bent and crippled, supported by a cane. And at last, a lifeless skeleton. Kuang Shi shuddered.

The touch of someone's hand on his shoulder startled him and made him spin around, only to face a young man with a shaved head, orange robes, and two vertical lines of clay marking his forehead. Kuang Shi recognized him as one of the Hare Krishna devotees, whom he had seen on campus from time to time. He heard that they even gave regular *yoga* classes, or something like that. With his busy schedule Kuang Shi never thought to attend any of their programs.

"What do you think?" the young man asked. "Do you

find the exhibit interesting?"

"It's pretty impressive. Must have taken you a while to put it all together. You've shown the changes in a person's life pretty nicely. I'm studying biochemistry, and I've been looking at these very changes your exhibit portrays on the level of cellular interactions."

"Well, if you're a scientist you're probably aware of the fact that nearly all the cells in your body are replaced every seven years."

"Not the brain cells," Kuang Shi corrected him.

The young American devotee smiled at the point. "Okay, but at least you'd have to admit that within this man's life of some seventy years, his body undergoes constant changes, cells and tissue being replaced continuously. So the body at death is certainly not the same one that one had at birth; yet no one could say that it's a different person with each bodily alteration."

"I can grant you that," Kuang Shi admitted.

"There's just one person, but it's his body that changes repeatedly throughout life. This is very nicely explained in an ancient book called the *Bhagavad-gītā*, which gives an appropriate example:

> As a person puts on new garments, giving up old ones, the soul similarly accepts new material bodies, giving up the old and useless ones.

"In other words, changing our clothes does not change the body. Do you follow?" Kuang Shi nodded. "The point is that the self within is not basically affected by all these changes. That's the purpose of this 'Changing Bodies' exhibit."

Kuang Shi's scientific training made him skeptical. What place did superstitious ideas like the existence of a soul in the body have in the modern world of science and reason? Moreover, the young man's dress reminded him of the Buddhist monks in his own country, who had lost all importance in the light of scientific discoveries about the real nature of things. Festival of India? Well . . . just look what's happened to India, he thought, because of all its religious sentiment.

"Just what is this *soul?*" Kuang Shi asked. "The body has a brain which performs the function of thinking. The thoughts and impressions are stored within the brain and form a constant link as the body changes. There's no reason to believe in a soul."

Their conversation had begun to attract some curious bystanders who had been looking at the same exhibit. Kuang Shi had no interest to continue if it meant he would have to make a spectacle of himself in some sort of public debate. The young devotee was smiling, as if he found Kuang Shi's concept somehow amusing. Kuang Shi didn't, but before he could turn to leave, the young man startled him by speaking out even more loudly, as if he wanted to be heard by everyone now gathered around them.

"There's an important scientific difference between the body and the soul. You're a scientist, you should know this." Kuang Shi felt both embarrassed and proud. The devotee directed their attention to the appropriate figures in the exhibit. "The body is born, it grows, it stays, it produces by-products, then it begins to decay, and at the last stage it vanishes. Therefore, the body is a nonpermanent material thing. However, the body's proprietor—the soul—is different."

"Has anyone ever seen the soul?" asked an elderly businessman who had joined the group of listeners.

"Has anyone ever seen his mind? Has anyone seen his intelligence?" came the devotee's swift response. From behind his steel-rimmed glasses the young man's eyes seemed to dance, as if to provoke his listeners into a discussion. Kuang Shi was not about to allow science to be bettered by some superstitious nonsense.

"What is your *proof* of the soul?" he blurted out.

"The *proof* of the soul is consciousness," the young man said coolly, satisfied that he had provoked the challenge. Kuang Shi wished that he had remained aloof, but having committed himself to the debate he was bound to defend himself personally as well as the position of material science. He listened attentively, trying to find some mistake or inconsistency in the young man's reasoning.

"Consciousness is the symptom of the soul. Although the soul cannot be seen with the material eyes, because it is not material, its existence can be understood through the symptom of consciousness. Today it's cloudy. Although we cannot see the sun, no one doubts its presence beyond the clouds. Why?" The crowd was silent. "Why?" he repeated.

"Because of the sunlight," someone answered offhandedly from somewhere in the swelling crowd.

"Who said that?"

A young student, perhaps a freshman in college, stepped forward, somewhat shyly. The devotee now directed his attention to the student. "Okay, right. Just as the sunshine indicates the presence of the sun, consciousness in the body reveals the presence of the soul. Do you follow?"

Before the Krishna devotee could intimidate the young student, Kuang Shi interrupted, "This explanation is not at all convincing. There's no need to postulate the existence of a soul. The body is alive, and therefore it is conscious."

"The body is dead, not alive!" The audience snickered at the devotee's feisty reply as the debate warmed up.

"See that automobile? Can it drive itself? It can move if a person turns on the engine. Otherwise, it's an inert machine, just dead matter. Our bodies are also machines—let's say, vehicles for our souls. Because the soul is within the body, the body moves and appears to be alive, and when the soul leaves the body at the time of death, the body loses all consciousness and stops moving, just like a machine whose engine has been turned off. It's simple."

"Wait a minute," Kuang Shi interjected. "According to science, life is a sequence of coordinated chemical reactions producing progressively more complex building blocks, like DNA, RNA, then amino acids, then cells, and ultimately human beings. Life is built from material elements, just like these buildings all around us."

"But the buildings were built by someone. So who builds our bodies?" the devotee replied.

"You should know that scientists have already succeeded in synthesizing genes, amino acids, and other substances which are the building blocks of life."

"But buildings are not alive. It's people who live in them who are the *real* life. You're a scientist, perhaps you'd like to answer this question: Can you manufacture a chicken egg in your laboratory? You can analyze each part of the egg: the hard outside shell, the soft white layer, the yellow yolk in the center, and so on. I doubt you'd have any problems with that. It's probably simple chemically. My question is this: Starting with the chemicals, can you combine them together to produce a chicken egg?"

The audience's silence made the oddity of the question echo strangely in Kuang Shi's ears. He strained for an answer, but nothing came. It seemed easy enough . . . a *chicken* egg? He pondered, but nothing came.

"Well, maybe we can't do it yet," he stuttered, "but in the future I know we'll be able to."

"In the *future*!" mocked the young devotee. "My dear scientist, don't you know the famous saying, 'Trust no future no matter how bright'? Go to a store without any money and try to purchase something by promising to pay for it in the future. Who'll trust you?"

The laughter that broke out in the crowd struck Kuang Shi's ears like a clap of thunder. He barely heard the devotee conclude, "So, until you can manufacture an egg in your lab, the chicken is a better scientist than you!" Practically everyone laughed, and Kuang Shi turned red. It didn't matter that the crowd now began to disperse and that they would probably never meet him again. It was the *principle* of the thing that disturbed him. How could he, a Ph.D. in biochemistry, be defeated by a junior in both age and education? Kuang Shi had always been proud of his intelligence, it had rarely let him down. He was not accustomed to being stymied—all over a chicken egg! He felt humiliated, but *why?* He blinked. The devotee was looking him right in the eye, smiling, but without malice. Kuang Shi searched his eyes, but could find no trace of derision.

"My name is Ananta," he said warmly, offering his hand. "I hope you're not offended." As a matter of fact, he was, but he replied politely, "No."

"Good. I didn't mean to. It's obvious that you're well educated and could no doubt understand the scientific basis of our philosophy, given some study."

"Philosophy? *What* philosophy?" he snorted, though the flattery helped to ease his hurt feelings.

"Are you from Japan?" the young man asked. Kuang Shi could not remember the number of times in the last five years that people had confused his nationality. In the beginning it had infuriated him, but he no longer felt bothered. "No, I'm from China."

"China? Really? That's great!" Americans always seemed impressed to meet someone from China, as if it were some sort of mysterious and unknown world. They were always so curious to meet someone actually born there. Yet Ananta's enthusiasm was somehow different.

"My spiritual master has visited China many times, and he speaks of it often, of what he believes could be the Chinese people's great destiny."

Kuang Shi was astonished. What did this philosophy, *whatever* it was, have to do with China? Most intriguing. He wondered what this "great destiny" was. Political? Sociological? Some sort of economics? And what on earth could any of these have to do with chicken eggs? He was tempted to pursue the point when it suddenly occurred to him that nearly half an hour had slipped by.

"I really do have to go. I'm late as it is for dinner," he said, excusing himself. It was past six and he still had nearly an hour to go to reach his Uncle Lawrence's house at the far end of Queens. This much was certain: he was not going to risk being late for Aunt Shiao Lin's great cooking just to debate chicken egg philosophy.

"Wait! Here, take this." Before he could refuse him, the young devotee thrust a small book into Kuang Shi's hand.

Kuang Shi wasn't interested in buying any book, especially some kind of a strange philosophy book. He was feeling bolder. "Great destiny of China" indeed!

Ananta reassured him, "It's a gift. Just promise me you'll read it. It was written especially for scientists. Can we meet again?"

"I'm very busy. Thank you for the gift. I'll try to look it over."

"By the way, my spiritual master will be here at the exhibition all day tomorrow, and since it's Saturday, you're probably not working."

Kuang Shi admired the young man's persistence.

"We'll see. I can't promise anything." Kuang Shi had no real intention of coming back just to be tricked again. Chicken eggs!

3

AS THE CROWDED UNDERGROUND train sped toward the borough of Queens, the residential area for many New Yorkers who worked in the city, Kuang Shi tried to sit comfortably, feeling himself lucky to have gotten a window seat. It was six-twenty, still rush hour, and the train was packed tightly with secretaries, businessmen, and workers eager to escape the congestion of Manhattan and get to their more peaceful residences in Queens. It was at such times that Kuang Shi was reminded of the teeming buses in Beijing, crowded to the point of suffocation. There, relatively fewer people rode the subway because it had such a limited route, unlike New Yorkers, who depended on the vast and sprawling subway network which linked the five boroughs of the city, much as the buses did in Beijing.

Kuang Shi smiled at the thought that Americans would probably have a fight if a passenger dared to shove another while boarding or leaving the train. In some respects his countrymen were far more tolerant, accepting such hardships as an inevitable part of life. On the other hand, his countrymen would never tolerate seeing their buses vandalized as New York subway trains were by gangs of youths who seemed compelled to fill every square inch of the outer and inner surfaces of the cars with wild scrawling graffiti. Painted designs were daubed, splashed, streaked everywhere. The result was unimaginable, barbaric, Kuang Shi thought. Riding a New York subway for the first time, a visitor to the city, try as he might, could never mistake all this paint for some kind of "abstract art." It was a complete vulgarization of words, names, and drawings, like a civilization gone mad. He wondered why the city authorities seemed incapable of controlling the situation. The Beijing police would certainly have taken immediate action. But then, Chinese people would never think of defacing public property so recklessly. It happened in the Cultural Revolution, but everyone admitted that that was pure madness. Although Americans had more than enough wealth (even a poor man here enjoyed a standard of living far beyond China's wealthy), there were far more crimes and other social ills. It was a great paradox, one Kuang Shi could not easily understand. On one hand he enjoyed the advantages of the West—its facilities, amenities, pleasures, and, yes, he had to admit to himself, its extraordinary liberties.

But, he thought, looking again at the wild paint-strewn subway car, there certainly were reasonable limits to liberty. Yet he knew that too many constraints frustrated the human spirit and stifled a nation's progress. China had already learned that bitter lesson. What to do? Kuang Shi absent-mindedly fingered the book he had received from the Krishna devotee.

Nearly half an hour remained before he reached the end of the line, where he would transfer to a bus. He looked at the title: *Easy Journey to Other Planets*, by His Divine Grace A. C. Bhaktivedanta Swami Prabhupāda. The cover depicted a *yogi* sitting in meditation. Kuang Shi immediately thought of Buddhism, perhaps because of the lotus flower designs. He looked at the portrait of the author on the back cover. It was hard to recognize his nationality. He looked very determined and kind.

He opened the book and read the dedication: "to the scientists of the world ..." The scientists of the world? What on earth did *yoga* and scientists have in common? Biochemistry ... birth ... death ... changing bodies. What was the connection? Kuang Shi rapidly reviewed the day's seemingly random episodes—the Ph.D. notice, the Festival of India, this stifling subway ride to Queens. Was there some pattern to all this? Kuang Shi's eyes returned to the book's title. What "easy journey"? He thumbed through the pages and came to the large section of color plates at the center of the book. He was struck by an illustrated version of the same exhibit he had just seen. "Changing Bodies." He read the caption:

> As the embodied soul continually passes, in this body, from boyhood to youth to old age, the soul similarly passes into another body at death. A sober person is not bewildered by such a change.

Another body? That's absurd. Death is final. There was reference to a page number; Kuang Shi turned to the text. He was trained to inquire and study in his research, and to reflect carefully on the findings before coming to a conclusion. To be fair-minded, he turned each page carefully. He approached the book with the same inquisitive eye he would have given a research paper in the science library, but he wasn't sure why he should in this case.

Before he knew it, the train had reached the last stop. He jumped up and moved with the flow of passengers up to street level and into the open air. The bus was waiting, all the seats fully occupied. He didn't mind standing; he had some things to think about.

Kuang Shi was not one to be emotional: He prided himself in being rational, even critical. Aloofly he had been analyzing the little book, withholding any final judgment. He looked at his watch and realized that he had only half an hour left and would have to study the rest of the book much more carefully. But the part that he had just read gave a pretty clear indication what he could expect from reading more.

The subject seemed to be the same thing that he and other scientists had been researching for so long: What, essentially, is life? The book seemed to share a common theme with certain disturbing challenges to a wholly mechanistic model of the universe that was being sounded from within the scientific community itself. The question was basically this: How should science deal with consciousness? How can it be quantified and reduced to a formula to fit in with the other grand formulae of Einstein, Heisenberg, and Schrodinger, etc., which formed the basis of modern physics and cosmology? It had actually tantalized him often in his own work, because there certainly was no chemical formula for consciousness. What, indeed, *is* consciousness? Kuang Shi wondered, again fingering the book, if this wasn't the same thing as asking what life is. He flashed back to his meeting with the Krishna devotee. Changing bodies. Chicken eggs. Why *can't* a chicken egg be synthesized? Here he was, a doctoral candidate in biochemistry, and he had to admit that the devotee had stumped him.

He began to reflect a little more seriously on what the book said about these things. He tried to summarize what struck him as its main points. The author kept talking about an anti-material particle and insisted it was the source of consciousness. There was even an anti-material universe. Kuang Shi humorously wondered if that might not be the same thing that Stephen Hawking at Cambridge meant when he mysteriously alluded to a white-hole universe on the other side of a black hole?

This much of it he could possibly handle, but the conclusion the book was apparently moving toward—a supreme anti-material *being?*—that surely was science fiction. Yet Kuang Shi wasn't so sure, especially since the author was proposing what sounded like a rather practical method for understanding anti-matter. *Yoga.* He pulled back. Where was this all leading? Could the practice of *yoga* really lead to such knowledge? And had anyone ever seen this anti-material particle? Even traveled to the anti-material world and returned to talk about it? A supreme being? The questions tossed around in Kuang Shi's mind.

He had always trusted science because it yielded predictable results based on experiments. Like other scientists, he had been studying the complex structures and properties of matter—electrons, atoms, and whole gamut of sub-atomic particles. But the author of this book appeared to say that they were uncovering only half-truths, while ignoring the anti-material dimension—the basis of consciousness and therefore life itself. Kuang Shi was well aware of the limitations of the mechanistic approach. Nearly all scientists accepted the fact that there were still troubling questions that remained unanswered in practically every field of science. Though scientists had been speculating for millennia, there were still no proven ideas as to the origin of the universe. Many of the most popular proposals directly contradicted each other. Besides, it struck him, how could one be sure that three hundred years from now these very theories would not seem as absurd to the people of the future as the flat earth idea does to us, or the notion only a few hundred years ago that earth was the center of the solar system?

Researchers into the origins of life, biochemists like himself, were in as much confusion as their counterparts in other fields. Darwin's theory provided the first proweful paradigm of evolution. Since then most have accepted that life could have come about from purely physical processes: electrons and protons interacting with one another and gradually coming together to form more and more complicated forms—from the simplist to the most complex, the human species. Yet dispite its common acceptance, the premise of Darwin's theory was not a proven, irrefutable law. Heisenberg's principal only admitted the "uncertainty" of measuring everything in motion, and even Einstein could not come up with his much yearned-for unified field theory. Kuang Shi realized almost with shock that for lack of a better explanation, what to speak of proof, scientists ascribed to the belief, more or less, that the original cause of everything was nothing more than some principle of grand cosmic chance. Kuang Shi laughed. The young devotee's statement, "The chicken is a better scientist than you are" had sounded unfair, but now he found it amusing. So many missing links, so many scientists scratching their heads, bewildered. Heisenberg might be correct after all, in a way he didn't expect. This alternately tickled and puzzled Kuang Shi.

He looked around at the other passengers in the bus and then stared out the window into the night, absorbed in his thoughts. Passengers nodded in and out of sleep, while a few talked to their fellow travelers. He doubted whether any ever gave much thought to the ideas he was contemplating. They left such matters to the scientists without realizing how much these basic issues affected the way they viewed themselves, their decisions, their feelings, their relationships, their behavior—in fact, every aspect of their life.

For Kuang Shi, being a scientist meant much more than simply performing experiments on mice or monkeys. He was about to be awarded a Ph.D., and he wanted to take his degree not merely to enhance his prestige but to prepare himself for greater responsibilities, whatever they might be. It was here, on this point, that his Chinese upbringing, especially his father's training, was influential. A scientist could be a very important servant of the public. It was this sense of larger commitment that was prompting Kuang Shi to think about what this little book was saying. The ideas were startling. If it could be proven, somehow, scientifically, that life arose from something more than just a chemical soup, that inside the body there was something life-giving, something that wasn't at all material ... What *was* that thing at the ultimate source of it all? And this book left no doubt—it suggested an experiment which was so easy that anyone could perform it. It boggled the mind. If it were true, even theoretically, the accepted foundation of knowledge would be shaken in a way no economic, social, or political revolution had ever previously done. And he, Li Kuang Shi, Ph.D., could be at the forefront of it all.

The bus finally reached Forest Hills, a prestigious residential area for New York's upper middle-class, and stopped two blocks from his uncle's home. As he exited, Kuang Shi inhaled the fresh air—one of the many benefits of living in suburban Queens. His head cleared of all weighty thoughts. He liked the homes in Forest Hills, each architecturally unique and situated on a quarter-acre plot. Although it was still too early for flowers, the hedges, trees, and gardens were neatly manicured. Every family had at least two cars, and some had as many as three or four.

His uncle, Chung Shi Loong, or Lawrence Chung, the name he had adopted soon after his arrival in New York City in 1950, had not always enjoyed such opulence. He had boarded a freighter and made the journey from Hong Kong as a cook's helper and immediately found work washing dishes fifteen hours a day in a Chinese restaurant. He lived frugally, saving every penny. Compared with other Americans, he was impoverished. But Lawrence Chung didn't mind, because his life had vastly improved over what it was in Hong Kong, what to speak of China! His thrift paid off: within five years he had saved enough to open a small Chinese restaurant. He named it Jade Mountain, and it soon gained a reputation for good but inexpensive food.

He was thirty-five years old when in 1965, his marriage with Shiao Lin was arranged. Both their families were originally from Guangzhou, and although Shiao Lin had been living as a refugee in Hong Kong, the marriage arrangements were made by their respective relatives.

Unlike her adaptable husband, Shiao Lin had difficulty adjusting to America. She refused to change her name and at first held tightly to many Chinese ways. But she was a hard worker and with her help their fortunes greatly improved. Within a matter of years he was able to open a second restaurant, and with the profits from the two establishments moved from the small dingy apartment in Chinatown to a new home in Forest Hills.

Now 38 years after Lawrence's arrival, their days of struggle were now far behind. Their children, Kuang Shi's cousins, Johnny (named after the late president John F. Kennedy) and Susan, enjoyed the full benefits that middle-class America provided. Lawrence Chung wanted his children to grow up as typical Americans, just like the neighbor's kids next door. Shiao Lin at last gave up all hope of preserving any Chinese traditions. Now, apart from their Oriental features, there was no way to tell Johnny and Susan apart from their other friends. Their tastes and interests were nearly one hundred percent American, and they felt a little awkward when asked about China. Except for some household words, greetings, and proverbial sayings, they didn't speak much Chinese at home and remained pretty much ignorant of most traditions.

Kuang Shi admired his uncle for being progressive, optimistic, and above all determined. But sometimes he felt a little disturbed by Johnny and Susan's indifference to their Chinese background. When he had first arrived from China they had laughed at his typically Chinese ways. They criticized his plain dress and his faltering English.

Although they were merely having a good time at his expense, Kuang Shi took their ridicule seriously. He purchased stylish clothing and paid a fellow student to coach him in English.

Kuang Shi was equally amused by his cousins' habits. For example, their predilection for chewing gum. But what most surprised him was their lack of proper respect for their parents. Uncle Larry, as his uncle insisted on being called, with his easygoing friendly nature, had helped Kuang Shi through this difficult period of adjustment. And Shiao Lin, in the absence of her elder sister, Kuang Shi's mother, showered him with motherly affection. They both insisted that he spend Sundays with them, and for the first two years he dutifully made the hour and a half journey to Queens. When his weekends filled up with studies, he stayed in touch by phone, though he still managed to visit them at least once a month.

It was Susan who answered when he rang the door bell. "It's Charlie!" she yelled out. "Charles" was the name his uncle had selected for him because he felt it had a distinguished, gentlemanly, European sound. Kuang Shi had no reason to doubt his uncle's advice, but as it turned out, most preferred to address him by the more familiar "Charlie." Either was preferable to Americans who became easily confused by his Chinese name.

"Charlie! Come on in!" his uncle called out jovially from the living room. Susan took Kuang Shi's light jacket and hung it in the closet. As he walked through the hallway, he heard a baseball game blaring from the T.V. Lawrence reclined on a large easy chair, his feet propped upon a cushion, while his son Johnny sprawled out on one of the two sofas.

"Shiao Lin, Charlie's here. How's everything, Charlie?" he asked, his eyes still glued to the set. He was a big sports fan, and it was hard for him to withdraw his attention from the T.V.

His aunt was genuinely pleased to see him. "Kuang Shi, I'm so happy to see you," she said affectionately. "It's been a long time since you stayed overnight with us."

"Sit down," said Uncle Lawrence, his attention still riveted to the TV. "Johnny, will you please make some room for your cousin?" Johnny only slightly adjusted himself.

"You know he doesn't like baseball," said Shiao Lin. "Kuang Shi, come in the kitchen and keep me company." He was happy to follow her. It was true, he did find baseball boring. "Guess what we're having for dinner. Wonton, one of your favorite dishes. Your mother loved the way I made it, and at times like this you remind me of her," she said.

Shiao Lin studied her nephew for a moment. Except for his stocky build and broad shoulders, which he had inherited from his father, he had his mother's smooth complexion, full eyebrows, and brilliant white teeth. These features, combined with his affable yet serious nature, made association with him as pleasantly enjoyable for her as it did for almost everyone who met him.

"*Ni jingcháng raóguo* wo," Kuang Shi smiled, pleased by his aunt's affection. He took a seat at the table while she attended to her cooking.

"Can I help?"

"You'll never guess what happened this week," Shiao Lin continued, as if she hadn't heard him. "Susan was accepted as a cheerleader at high school."

"That's great!" he said somewhat mechanically.

"She'll be starting practice next fall."

"Practice?" inquired Kuang Shi absentmindedly.

"Practicing *cheerleading* of course," she replied, looking over at her nephew. "You're not listening. Something's on your mind. I know you well enough. Out with it. What's the secret?"

Kuang Shi smiled. "My Ph.D. thesis has been accepted," he said, although other things were occupying his mind.

Shiao Lin put aside the pot she was stirring. "What?!" Astonished, she replied, "And you've kept it a secret? What a wonderful surprise! And no one knows it yet?" She nodded in the direction of the living room.

"You're the very first," said Kuang Shi, delighted by his aunt's genuine happiness for him. It picked him up and helped dispel his introspective mood.

Without a moment's delay, Shiao Lin took him by the arm and marched into the sitting room. She walked up to the T.V. and stood in front of it, blocking everyone's view.

"Shiao Lin, what are you doing!" Lawrence was obviously annoyed.

Kuang Shi could hardly contain his laughter as he watched his aunt, to everyone's amazement, turn off the set.

"Mom, what are you doing!" Johnny cried out.

"Shiao Lin, what the . . . ?" Uncle Lawrence was in complete disbelief. He had never seen his wife do anything like this before.

"Kuang Shi has a surprise for us," she said, calmly smiling. "Tell them, Kuang Shi," she urged.

Kuang Shi looked over at his uncle and cousins. "They've accepted my dissertation."

"What! When? Why didn't you tell us? Charlie, are you serious?" Uncle Lawrence sat up.

"Of course he is," said Shiao Lin.

Within a moment Lawrence was on his feet embracing his nephew. "This is the happiest moment of my life," he said, nearly in tears. "Charlie, I can't believe it!"

"And why not?" said his wife happily. "Do you think our nephew is ordinary?"

"Of course not! He's brilliant. He's going to win the Nobel Prize. Charlie—or should I say Dr. Li?"

"Wait 'til Mrs. Yang hears the news," joked Susan. "She'll want to arrange her daughter's marriage with Charlie immediately."

"Stop teasing your cousin," Shiao Lin told her daughter.

"That's not the only news, Uncle," said Kuang Shi. "I've received an offer from a second pharmaceutical company—Abbott Laboratories—one of the biggest in the country."

"How much? Come on! Tell us how much they've offered?"

Kuang Shi was silent, smiling, increasing the suspense. He knew that his uncle tended to measure success in dollars and cents. "Make a guess," he said.

The room grew still, broad smiles on everyone's face. Larry Chung squinted, knitting his brow, and thought for a moment, then blurted out, "Seventy thousand!" Kuang Shi shook his head. "More?" Kuang Shi nodded and his uncle's smile broadened even more. "Eighty thousand?" Kuang Shi pointed his finger upward. "Ninety thousand!" said Uncle Lawrence, as if counting every dollar.

"One hundred thousand dollars a year!" Kuang Shi grinned and raised his eyebrows. Lawrence's pleasure seemed boundless, and Shiao Lin cried. Susan leaped up and down as if cheering her high school team to victory, and even Johnny seemed genuinely excited.

"Have you informed your father and mother yet?" said Shiao Lin between her husband's excited exclamations. "We should call them right now."

"I'm going to phone the whole world," laughed Lawrence Chung. "This calls for a celebration. There's nothing good enough for a nephew as special as you. I'm going to hold the biggest banquet that Chinatown has ever seen." He walked over to the telephone and dialed the restaurant. "Is Eddie there? It's Larry. Hello, Eddie? Get the reservation book! Is the Emperor Room full tomorrow night?" After a moment: "Hmmm, they'll understand. Move them downstairs. I want it for the entire evening. We're going to throw the biggest party you've ever seen. Tell Feng and Wu to come real early tomorrow morning to start preparing. They're to give special attention to the Eight Treasures Pudding and the Suckling Pig, and tell them to go down to Fulton Street and pick the fish themselves. My nephew Charlie's about to get the Nobel Prize!" Kuang Shi protested, but his uncle merely waved him off. "He's been awarded a Ph.D. degree. I'll call you back later." Lawrence Chung hung up the phone. "I'm going to invite everyone I know for this. It isn't every immigrant who can boast of a nephew with a doctorate from Columbia."

Kuang Shi savored the family's euphoria. After five years of effort he deserved to feel a little satisfied. He had always pushed aside thoughts of fame and wealth, but now, for a moment, he relished the praise. It felt good. In fact, he too wanted to celebrate.

4

IT WAS NEARLY NOON, and the brilliant rays of the overhead sun stimulated the swarms of shoppers thronging Fifth Avenue. Kuang Shi shared their buoyant mood, reveling in the warmth of the fine spring day. The freshness of the season created a feeling of expectation, a promise of things to come. At least for Kuang Shi, the day held great hope. Judging by his uncle's mood the previous night, he knew that there were sure to be dozens of specially prepared dishes and wine flowing without limit.

He was free until evening, and his uncle's high spirits-had been infectious. Coming back to Manhattan, he had ridden the subway train an extra two stops just to enjoy the walk up Fifth Avenue. There was no other street like it in New York, certainly not Beijing's Chan An nor Wang Fu Jin Streets. There was nothing comparable to it anywhere else in America, perhaps the whole world. In its grand proportions, beginning with magnificent Washington Square Arch to the northern end of Central Park, Fifth Avenue contained within its one hundred city blocks the most stately, elegant, and important buildings in New York City. On days like this, Kuang Shi would walk the entire length at a stretch, enjoying the exercise and the relief from his studies. He had become familiar with the Avenue's main attractions, having seen them often in five years. North from Washington Square he would pass New York University and soon come to his favorite book shop. Strands, where he had found many useful and delightful secondhand books. Kuang Shi mused on the good fortune of Americans, to be able to avail themselves of any book on any subject they were interested in. The educated Chinese people were also avid readers, and as the literacy rate increased, there was a growing demand for books on all subjects. Yet, he recalled ruefully, all too often books were unavailable, due either to government policies or simply to shortage of supply. It was not uncommon for a book to sell out on the first day of its release.

Everything on Fifth Avenue would amaze his countrymen, as it still did him. The heights were breathtaking, and one felt insignificant against massive skyscrapers of brick, marble, steel, and glass. None could equal in size the one hundred two stories of the Empire State Building, in beauty the Gothic St. Patrick's Cathedral, or for popularity Rockefeller Center. Further on one came to the garment district, then fashionable department stores selling diamond necklaces worth one million dollars and children's trains costing more than five thousand dollars, prices unimaginable to a man who earned a mere one hundred *yuan* a month. But not in America, where the average income was nearly twenty thousand dollars, and especially not in New York, where millionaires were not uncommon.

Suddenly, the pulsating shriek of a siren filled the air, and an ambulance rushing on Fifth Avenue halted abruptly a block ahead of Kuang Shi. He quickened his pace, but by the time he reached the scene a crowd had gathered and medics were carrying a stretcher to the ambulance. Kuang Shi looked quickly at the building, a bank, and then back at the stretcher just as the ambulance doors were opening to admit the form of a middle-aged man neatly dressed in a grey business suit. The crowd was already thinning when a bank officer emerged from the building and said, "Heart attack, I bet. Boy! He went just like *that*!" And snapped his fingers so sharply that the sound broke clean through the din of the New York midday noise and ricocheted off Kuang Shi's ears. "Just like that," he murmured to himself, almost numbly. Feeling a little queasy, he quickly separated himself from the scene, as if the distance of another city block would protect him from a similar fate. He busied himself looking into shop windows, trying to ignore the siren as the screaming ambulance sped into the distance. Just like that!

He eased up. An unfamiliar anxiety began to cloud the cheerfulness of the day. In the bank. On the stretcher. Just like that. Changing bodies? Birth, death. And then? An easy journey to other planets?

The unspoken anxiety now began to take shape as a tangible fear and work its way upward from his gut to lodge in his throat. He winced and swallowed hard, trying to digest the dread. "I'm glad it wasn't me!" he cried out. Fighting back tears, feeling alone in the crowd, a haunting whisper repeated itself, "I don't want to die, I don't want to die!" It was an unfamiliar voice, yet it belonged to something very close. For a person always very certain about everything he did, Kuang Shi now felt confused. He stopped. He stared blankly ahead, his vision turned within. With the greatest effort he asked himself, "If I am only a bunch of chemicals, why am I so afraid? Do chemicals cry? Maybe there is something else." He looked down at his trembling hands. There's got to be something else, but no answer came. Suddenly, he looked up. Fifty-ninth Street and Central Park South. He looked left. Just barely visible in the distance multicolored tenting flapped in the April breeze. One thing was certain, the rest of his afternoon would be spent with the Krishna devotees.

Ananta had been practicing *yoga* since he was fifteen years old, attracted by its healthy outlook and natural lifestyle. Only after meeting a Krishna teacher in his freshman year at college did he realize that there was more to it than exercises and bodily postures. He began to study *yoga* philosophy and quickly adjusted his whole life to conform to the teachings. By his junior year he had already considered a career as a *yoga* instructor, and in keeping with tradition he wore light orange robes symbolizing renunciation. He explained to his parents that the *yoga* dress served the same purpose as a policeman's uniform or a doctor's smock: easy identification for those in need of their help.

As Kuang Shi made his way toward the Festival of India, a large crowd watched as Ananta lay flat on his back and gradually raised his legs, arching them over his head until his toes rested on the ground. All this had been accomplished within a single inhalation of breath.

"This is called the 'plow' pose," he explained. "Nerves and muscles are strengthened and the spine is kept flexible. This is the key to youthfulness. For those of you who are getting stiff spines, be careful—it's a sign of old age. Besides invigorating and toning up the nerves, muscles, thighs, pelvis, abdomen, and the heart, it prevents the loss of appetite—*and*, it can cure constipation and diabetes. Let's do the headstand next." With full concentration he lifted his body with folded knees until he was upside down, supporting himself on his head and elbows with perfect ease. The audience, however, applauded the performance more as a gymnastic feat than as a way to control the senses and the mind, the real goal of *yoga*.

Someone in the audience shouted, "Let's see you fly!" People laughed. Smiling, Ananta quickly replied, "Actually, ancient *yogis* did have such powers. Not only could they fly, they walked on water, lived for weeks without breathing. They were able to acquire anything they liked simply by their will." More laughter. "Yes, we laugh," Ananta added, just as Kuang Shi walked up to hear him conclude, "but *yoga* has something much greater to offer. Modern science has already achieved much of what *yoga* could accomplish." *Yoga* and science, hmmm. I got here just in time, he thought. Kuang Shi wanted to hear more.

"So what *is* the real purpose of *yoga*? The word itself comes from Sanskrit and means 'to connect,' to concentrate the mind on the self within instead of our ever-changing bodies." Changing bodies. The vivid memory of the corpse in the grey flannel suit flashed before Kuang Shi.

Ananta directed their attention to the "Changing Bodies" exhibit, where his spiritual master, Sanatan Swami, stood speaking to a crowd of perhaps two hundred people. "I'd like to invite all of you to accompany me to our 'Changing Bodies' exhibit and meet my teacher, who is a great master of *yoga*." Kuang Shi moved with the others toward the tall form of Ananta's teacher.

In their first meeting Sanatan Swami had delivered a lecture to teachers and students at Ananta's college and had taken a special interest in him, sensing his sincere interest in *yoga*. Sanatan Swami was much more than an ordinary college professor. He was greatly learned, and what made his erudition so special was the way in which he combined a mastery of many disciplines into a profound, consistent world view. His philosophy of life was not the mere product of a fertile imagination nor limited to his personal experiences, although these were certainly varied and great. His pride was to uphold the ancient teachings of an unbroken line of spiritual masters extending back thousands of years. He had an unshakable faith in the wisdom of his predecessors and saw himself as their humble servant. His purpose was not to try to excel them by adding something new, but to represent their realizations in the light of modern scientific knowledge. Sanatan Swami had therefore dedicated himself to a life of service. He lived simply and austerely and made no selfish efforts for his own enjoyment. Ananta watched his spiritual master, senses perfectly under control, respond expertly to challenges from the large audience. He cherished occasions like today, because his spiritual master came into public and taught anyone even vaguely interested, offering priceless wisdom to all. As Ananta looked over the crowd, he suddenly saw Kuang Shi, who was intently observing the imposing form of the American Swami. He was large, over six feet tall, and Kuang Shi guessed his age to be about fifty or fifty-five. He was impressed by the Swami's forcefulness, yet he seemed very refined, especially the gestures he made in emphasizing a point, it struck Kuang Shi. His shaven head and orange robes gave him a Buddha-like dignity.

Kuang Shi was pleased by Ananta's friendly greeting. "I enjoyed your *yoga* demonstration," he told the young devotee. "Have you heard of Chinese *qigong*? There are many similarities." Ananta merely shook his head, and both turned again to listen to the lecture.

Sanatan Swami was replying to a question from a young lady who wanted to know how and *where* the soul could possibly live on after the body dies.

"This subject," Sanatan Swami explained, "has been elaborately described in the ancient dialogue called *Bhagavad-gītā*. It's originally written in the Sanskrit language, and it analyzes the science of the soul." He held up a copy of the book. "This edition is called *Bhagavad-gītā As It Is*. It was translated with commentary by His Divine Grace A.C. Bhaktivedānta Swami Prabhupāda." What he said next, Kuang Shi guessed, must have been Sanskrit. It sounded like beautiful and ancient poetry:

> na jāyate mriyate vā kadācin
> nāyaṁ bhūtvā bhavitā vā no bhūyaḥ
> ajo nityaḥ śāśvalo 'yaṁ purāṇo
> na hanyate hanyamāne śarīre

"What's he saying?" Kuang Shi whispered to Ananta. "Be patient, he'll give the translation in a minute."

> For the soul there is neither birth nor death at any time. He has not come into being, does not come into being, and will not come into being. He is unborn, eternal, ever-existing and primeval. He is not slain when the body is slain.
>
> The soul can never be cut to pieces by any weapon, nor burned by fire, nor moistened by water, nor withered by the wind.
>
> This individual soul is unbreakable and insoluble, and can be neither burned nor dried. He is everlasting, present everywhere, unchangeable, immovable and eternally the same.

"Finally," Sanatan Swami concluded, "it is said that the

soul is invisible, inconceivable, and immutable. These are all descriptions from the *Bhagavad-gītā*. Unlike the body, which requires air, light, and food, the soul requires none of these. As for your question, therefore, where the soul lives or, in other words, where the soul goes when it leaves the body—that is also explained in the *Bhagavad-gītā*." Sanatan Swami again quoted in Sanskrit and gave the translation:

> The living entity in the material world carries different conceptions of life from one body to another as the air carries aromas. Thus he takes one kind of body and again quits it to take another. The foolish cannot understand how a living entity can quit his body, nor can they understand what sort of body he enjoys under the spell of the modes of nature. But one whose eyes are trained in knowledge can see all this.

Some in the audience snickered or simply cocked their heads warily at what to them sounded strange and unbelievable. Sanatan Swami was not surprised by their response, for he knew that to them the idea of another birth was merely fantasy or at best a wishful dream. The science of reincarnation was as amazing to someone in New York as it was to someone in London, Shanghai, or Tokyo. It would take time and the patient work of many dedicated teachers to make this information widely known, because without proper training in self-realization, how could they be expected to understand this knowledge? Already he had seen a marked improvement in America due to the distribution of millions of books on the subject.

"As odd as it may sound, over one third of all Americans *accept* the soul's taking another birth." Looking over his large sidewalk audience, he searched for one who might understand. The crowd had lost a few people, but those who were staying on seemed to be warming to Sanatan

Swami, perhaps in spite of themselves. Kuang Shi reflected on what he had just heard and then remembered the dedication in the little book he had looked through—"to the scientists of the world." He wondered if he knew what science was or wasn't anymore. One thing he was fairly sure of, that Sanatan Swami was talking about a very special kind of science. For a brief moment he felt as though he were warily, unsurely making his way on a rope bridge high above a gorge, between two worlds, but the image was too disturbing and he shook it off immediately. He looked up again at Sanatan Swami and their eyes met. Kuang Shi felt reassured. The rope bridge steadied. Sanatan Swami noticed among the typical New York faces the particularly keen look of a young man whom he immediately recognized to be Chinese. Looking at him, he continued, "To help us understand the phenomenon of changing bodies . . ."

Kuang Shi's eyes widened. Why does this idea unsettle me so easily, he wondered, flashing again to the scene of the dead banker's body being unceremoniously carried off by the city ambulance.

". . . the *Bhagavad-gītā* cites this very nice example. Pure consciousness is like clean air: It carries different odors, some fragrant, some pungent. Similarly, consciousness becomes affected by whatever it comes in contact with. Thus, the conscious soul, when entering a particular body, identifies with that body, carrying the conception 'I am young,' 'I have become old,' 'I am a man,' 'I am a woman,' 'I am fat,' 'I am thin, white, black, American, European, Chinese, rich, poor.' In this way, one changes his body as he changes apartments—sometimes inhabiting a first-class residence, at other times a lower-class one." Kuang Shi smiled at the analogy. Now *that* makes sense. But if I'm not a scientist, and if I'm not Chinese, who am I?

"It's our consciousness which determines the body we inhabit, or in other words our next birth. Consciousness is such a powerful force, leading us here and there simply to fulfill our desires. And just as our desires determine our activities in this life, they also decide our future births. How this happens is described in the *Bhagavad-gītā*:

> Whatever state of being one remembers when he quits his body, O son of Kunti, that state he will attain without fail.

"This explains the process for changing one's body at the critical moment of death. Now, I know what many of you are thinking right now," Sanatan Swami added, "that one's future life hinges on but a moment's thought at death? Okay, let's analyze that last moment. Think of it in terms of using a calculator: When all the numbers you wanted added are entered, you press the 'total' button to get the final tally. In the same way, at the moment of death all the thoughts and actions of your entire lifetime are tallied up. Like King Bharat, for example, the emperor of the planet, who died while searching for his pet deer. His consciousness thus absorbed, he took a deer's birth."

This was too much for the audience. Sanatan Swami immediately checked their incredulity. "Look! You already accept the idea that humans have souls. Why are you so astonished and annoyed to hear that animals also have souls? It's very logical, isn't it?"

But their murmurs indicated that they weren't convinced.

"So, you think you're the only ones with souls?" he chided them. "Is that very reasonable? Don't you think that animals have consciousness? And what about birds and fish and plants?" He raised a finger to drive the point home. "That they are conscious is proof that they have souls. Not *only* are they conscious, they are also intelligent—perhaps not as intelligent as you, but intelligent nevertheless!"

"Fish have no intelligence!" shouted someone indignantly.

"Oh, not intelligent?" repeated the Swami, arching his eyebrows dramatically to show his wonder. Haven't you ever gone fishing? If you have, you'd never say a fish has no intelligence. You dangle some food before him, hoping he will bite on your hook. But nine times out of ten, he finds a way to get the food without being caught. That's intelligence!

"Even trees and plants have intelligence. If you build a wall next to where a tree is growing, the tree will grow around it. Somehow it will find the sunshine with its branches, the water with its roots. Without intelligence, how is this possible? Yes, I know what you're thinking," said Sanatan Swami anticipating their doubts. "But because other creatures are not as intelligent as humans doesn't mean that they have no intelligence. They are conscious beings just as we are spirit souls stuck within a material body.

"Let me tell you of a recent experience I had in India. I was living in a small village, where there were lots of domestic and wild animals roaming about. One day I made the mistake of leaving one of my books on a windowsill, and when I returned it was gone. I looked high and low for it; I even asked the family I was staying with: no one knew anything about it. But later that day someone knocked on the door to return my book. It seems that a monkey had stolen the book. Entering the fruit market, he had approached one of the vendors and offered it in exchange for some bananas. The vendor caught on to what the monkey had in mind and went along with the fun. When he realized it was in English, he brought it to me. So, you think that animals have no intelligence, no soul?"

Seeing how much the audience liked the story, Sanatan Swami made his final point. "*All* living entities have souls, but their intelligence and consciousness are not as developed as a human's. They use their intelligence merely to maintain their existence by eating, sleeping, mating, and defending. Humans, however, have highly developed intelligence, which sets them apart from others, and it is therefore most regrettable when human beings do little more with their life than exercise the same animal propensities—namely, eating, sleeping, mating, and defending. Human life is meant to understand the self, the difference between the soul and the body. A human being should *want* to know who he really is, where he originally comes from, what is the ultimate goal of life.

"The science of Krishna consciousness is meant to help find the answers to these questions, and such a science enables the soul to keep from being falsely identified with the body. So, when we regain our original pure consciousness, we will no longer be forced to accept another material birth, whether as a human, animal, or any other species. Instead, we shall be liberated from all material connections and return back to our original, eternal, all-knowledgeable, and fully blissful state. This should be our goal, everyone's goal, for it represents the perfection of human life."

Sanatan Swami looked with concern at his audience, hoping that it had grasped the few basic concepts he had tried to relay. There was no certainty when, if ever, he would again be seeing them. They had taken interest in the Festival of India as a passing curiosity, something to do in between their shopping or while visiting the park. He had held their attention as long as possible, but now they were becoming restless. Within minutes they would again be absorbed in temporary pursuits, forgetful of their eternal identity. Their ignorance pained him and in moments they would disperse. Seizing this final opportunity, he urged that they purchase one of the books which he now held aloft. He described each briefly: *Bhagavad-gītā*, the essence of all spiritual teachings; *Easy Journey to Other Planets; Coming Back*, scientific explanations of the soul's journey; and *Perfection of Yoga*. Some were interested and they came forward to purchase them. Ananta rushed forward to his spiritual master's side to assist in selling the books. Distributing transcendental literature gave Sanatan Swami the highest pleasure. Though they might forget his speech, books would make a lasting impression. Therefore his own spiritual master had stressed book distribution above all other activities.

Kuang Shi watched the crowd disperse in all directions. Quite a few drifted into the Festival's other exhibits. He soon stood alone at what had been the outer perimeter of the large audience. His solitary presence isolated him like an island, drawing Sanatan Swami's attention to him. They stood for a moment, silent, looking at one another. Despite Kuang Shi's shyness, Sanatan Swami's smile drew him magnetically.

Ananta was eager to introduce his new friend, knowing how important China was to his spiritual master. He quickly described their meeting the previous evening, but he fumbled when he realized he had forgotten to ask Kuang Shi his name. Kuang Shi volunteered, "My name is Charles Li. My friends call me Charlie."

"Charles?" questioned Sanatan Swami. "That's not your *real* name."

"No," admitted Kuang Shi, somewhat embarrassed, yet pleased. "My Chinese name is Li Kuang Shi."

"Ah, that's much nicer. 'Li Kuang Shi,' " repeated the teacher, fascinated to know its meaning.

The way in which Sanatan Swami carefully pronounced his name carried Kuang Shi back to his village home. He remembered his father, holding him on his lap, solemnly pronouncing, "Kuang Shi." Time and time again as he was growing up his father had reminded him that one day he must fulfill its meaning. Had his father known that he had changed his name, he would have been disappointed, even hurt.

" 'Kuang' means 'plenty' or 'wide' and 'Shi' means 'to give in charity.' Kuang Shi means 'to give in abundance.'" He spoke as if the words were meant for his father, hoping to reassure him by this explanation that he had not forgotten their intent.

"And how are you fulfilling such a glorious name?" beamed Sanatan Swami. Kuang Shi could only smile. Though there was practically no resemblance between the teacher and his father, the question could just as well have come from him.

"I'm afraid I haven't, and perhaps that is why I've changed my name," he excused himself sheepishly.

"The ancient Chinese culture was so much richer in comparison with our present American culture," began Sanatan Swami, launching into one of his favorite topics. "It would be a great shame if the last remains of that great culture were neglected and material advancement solely advocated. As one of the world's leading nations, China, like America, has a great destiny to fulfill."

"You sound like one of our Chinese leaders," Kuang Shi laughed. But he appreciated the point. America was sharing its technology with most of the world, and China, too, looked to the United States in so many ways. Certainly Kuang Shi had been benefitted personally. "America is the greatest nation," he said appreciatively.

But Sanatan Swami didn't fully share the young man's enthusiasm. He saw America's obsession with technology as both a blessing and as a curse. Certainly it provided man with ever new facilities, but without understanding life's ultimate goal these facilities could prove more dangerous than beneficial. As an uneducated child risks injury when playing with a sharpened knife, so a mankind unaware of life's ultimate purpose courts disaster while wielding technological advancement. It was a theme that would take time to explain. Looking at his watch Sanatan Swami suggested, "Why don't we have lunch together? I know a wonderful spot in the park, just beside the lake. Ananta. you remember—the grove of trees? We'll go on over there while you arrange lunch for the three of us. Let's have a picnic."

Kuang Shi had been planning not to eat lunch in order to make more room for the big dinner tonight at his uncle's restaurant. But it was hard to refuse his invitation. Besides, he wanted to spend the afternoon with them anyway. He didn't want to miss the opportunity to ask some questions of such a learned person. While Ananta went to make arrangements, Kuang Shi accompanied Sanatan Swami into the park.

5

THEY WERE AN UNUSUAL PAIR—the older American monk and the young Chinese scientist. They might have been more in character had their roles been reversed. A Chinese monk and an American scientist would have been truer to tradition, but blown by the winds of modern history, the seeds of divergent cultures had been transplanted in foreign soils, producing unusual social hybrids. For cosmopolitan New Yorkers, most of whom themselves were products of multiple cultures, the imposing presence of the tall American holy man along with his stocky Chinese friend went almost unnoticed. They had come to the park to be with their friends or families, to enjoy a leisurely Saturday afternoon. As Kuang Shi and the teacher passed through the park, some young boys skated by in precisioned maneuvers, showing off their skills on the smooth black pavement. The park was filled with a mass of humanity: lovers walking hand in hand, parents wheeling baby carriages, drunks sharing a bottle of wine, children running by with helium-filled balloons purchased at the nearby zoo, old men playing checkers on cement table boards, young Latino drummers and guitarists strumming different tunes, families picnicking, derelicts searching the garbage bins for discarded tin cans to earn a few pennies. In short, people of all sizes, shapes, ages, backgrounds, and interests had come together that spring day in Central Park. Walking paths, bicycle paths, horse paths, even the lake, dotted with colorful row-boats, were all filled with activity. Though the meadows and undulating hills were still nearly bald, no one seemed to mind the absence of grassy covering as they sat upon the hard brown earth enjoying the warmth of the noonday sun.

"Central Park always reminds me of Beijing's Purple Bamboo Park," Kuang Shi began. "The lake, boats, hills, even the weather is similar."

"But that park is *much* cleaner." injected Sanatan Swami. "And there is nice music playing over the loudspeakers."

"You've visited China?" Kuang Shi was surprised.

"Many times," smiled Sanatan Swami affably.

"Were you invited officially?"

"No," laughed the Swami. "I go simply as a tourist, to observe and study the place and its people. Nature is the greatest of teachers if you can simply learn to understand her language. We turn here." Kuang Shi followed the Swami over a small iron fencing that bordered the walkway. They had been circling the lake but now moved up a hillside into a wooded area. The parting bushes revealed an open space between a group of trees.

"In summer these trees form a canopy against the hot sun. It's one of my favorite spots. When I sit here I can forget the noise and pollution of this big city."

"But it seems that you're not the only one who knows about this place," said Kuang Shi, pointing at some discarded beer cans and the remnants of a camp fire. "Some drunkards no doubt. There are so many in New York."

"Or teenagers, or... who knows? Just about everyone drinks," said Sanatan Swami as he kicked the beer cans into the bushes and cleared a small area. Taking a plastic cloth from a shoulder bag, he proceeded to spread it over the ground. Removing his shoes, he sat down comfortably in cross-legged fashion. "There. That's better. You can sit here. Don't be shy. Take off your shoes."

"I prefer to keep them on, if I may." Kuang Shi sat down extending his legs forward, taking care that his shoes remained off the mat. "Your student said that you're a master of *yoga*," he said, appreciating the ease with which Sanatan Swami maintained what would have been to Kuang Shi a somewhat difficult sitting posture.

"Perhaps I know the kind of *yoga* you're thinking of. Last year when I visited China a young lady from Hawaii was teaching *yoga* on television." "Yes, one of my friends wrote me about it. They say that one can acquire superhuman powers."

"That's true," acknowledged the Swami. "But the real purpose of *yoga* is much deeper. Though the television show created an interest in *yoga*, it concentrated mostly on teaching the physical benefits only, without explaining the philosophy. Nearly everyone I met, when they understood that I practiced *yoga*, wanted me to demonstrate some bodily exercises. Some even wanted me to fly in the air."

Hoping to impress the teacher with his sincerity, Kuang Shi said, "I'm more interested to understand your beliefs.

There's something about them that intrigues me."

" 'Beliefs'?" repeated Sanatan Swami. "Perhaps that's not quite the word. You mean our philosophy? You may have your beliefs, I may have mine, but beliefs can be imperfect and subject to alteration. You may wonder why I'm rejecting the term 'beliefs.' It's because every living being in this world has four basic defects: His senses are imperfect, he makes mistakes, he becomes illusioned, and there is a tendency to be cheated and to cheat others. Under these circumstances we cannot really expect perfect knowledge from imperfect beliefs. Therefore let's talk on the basis of science rather than the beliefs of imperfect men."

That hit home. This is what he had come for. "Yes, I want to understand this idea of changing bodies scientifically. Last night I looked through the book given to me by your student."

"Which book?"

"*Easy Journey to Other Planets.* And I also heard your interesting speech today. I want to know if you can actually prove the existence of the soul and its journey from body to body. It sounds like nothing more than a theory to me. You say what you teach is scientific, but you have to be able to prove it by experiment."

Kuang Shi's pragmatic mind very much appealed to Sanatan Swami, who immediately took up the challenge.

"*Yoga* is a true science because it includes both theory and experimental proof. The basic theory is simple: Each of us is an eternal spiritual entity, different from this body. The body is made up of matter, but within it is an antimaterial particle which in Sanskrit is called *atma*, in English 'soul,' and in Chinese *líng hún*. It is this soul, or *líng hún*, that is actually alive. The body is dead matter energized by the soul."

"I'll concede the point theoretically. Please go on."

"Good. Let's proceed to the second principle: The universe is created and sustained by a supreme intelligent being."

"That's certainly a religious statement if I've ever heard one," Kuang Shi objected.

"Your education has prejudiced you to think in only one way without examining alternative ideas. That's not very scientific. You should be prepared to examine all theories with equal objectivity and draw your conclusions only at the end."

Kuang Shi was silent. It was true: he had never given the theory of creation any credence whatsoever. He continued to listen respectfully.

"Although materialistic scientists would have us believe that there is no supreme intelligent being, their denial isn't based on any evidence, nor have they any proof. There are many theories about how the universe began, but none has been in any way verified. However, the principle of a supreme being is eminently logical, and common sense leads us to this conclusion. After all, everything within our experience has a cause, doesn't it? Then why should we think the universe has none?" Sanatan Swami imitated the scientists, "'Chance. Pure chance. Nothing but chance. It's all random chance!' But," Sanatan Swami pointed his finger at Kuang Shi, "chance means they have no real answer to this question." Kuang Shi couldn't help but smile. "Take this wristwatch for example," he said, pulling his sleeve back. "How many components would you say are there in this watch?"

Kuang Shi hesitated, sensing that Sanatan Swami was trying to bait him with this seemingly harmless question.

"Take a guess," goaded the Swami. "How many pieces are in this watch? Three hundred? Five hundred? Well, how many?" he persisted.

"Perhaps a few hundred?" Kuang Shi finally conceded.

"Fine. Now let's take it apart, gathering the few hundred pieces in the palms of our hands." He made believe he had hundreds of pieces within his cupped palms and shook them. "Now let's shake these up and ... ," continuing, he threw the pieces high into the air. Sanatan Swami looked straight at Kuang Shi and paused for effect. "Now, what chance is there, when the pieces fall to the ground, that they will automatically form themselves into a wristwatch in perfect running order?"

Kuang Shi was silent. The answer was obvious. No chance at all.

But Sanatan Swami demanded an answer, "Well, what are the chances?"

"None," Kuang Shi admitted.

"Perhaps if we waited one year, or ten years, or a hundred, or a hundred million? Do you think that the pieces would eventually come together on their own?"

Kuang Shi was becoming impatient to get past the example. "No," he volunteered, "unless someone personally puts all the pieces together, they will never form a wristwatch on their own."

"Thank you. Applying the same logic, let's consider this universe where we cannot begin to estimate the number of components. Even in this small little hillside there are an incalculable number of atomic particles." He gestured to their surroundings. The sun poured through the bare branches, creating shadows of myriad variety. As Kuang Shi looked up at the trees and beyond to the sky and through the bushes to the lake which spread its way into the distance beyond his vision, he thought about the complexities of nature's creation. He stared down at the ground, at the earth, and tried to imagine how many countless molecules and atoms there were in even a square inch. Impossible. He looked up at the teacher and smiled.

"As a biochemist, you, much more than others, are fully aware of the precisioned order of nature's creation. The molecular machinery in a simple cell surpasses a modern city in complexity, and cells can reproduce themselves, something that no machine has ever been able to do. Just like the microcosmic cell, the macrocosmic universe is infinitely complex, yet moving in precisioned order." Sanatan Swami looked at Kuang Shi with the utmost sincerity. "Now, I ask you, in all honesty, can you imagine the creation to be the result of mere chance?"

Kuang Shi had indeed seen the point. Yet something within him fought against the inevitable conclusion. As a scientist he did admire nature's intricate design, but to acknowledge the existence of a so-called "supreme designer" was more than he was ready to admit.

"Just as in the electrical powerhouse there is the resident engineer," Kuang Shi knew what was coming next, "behind the universal creation there is the hand of a creator. As a scientist you should appreciate the fact that the *Bhagavad-gītā* is a verifiably scientific treatise. Just listen to a few quotations:

> Earth, water, fire, air, ether, mind, intelligence and false ego—all together these eight constitute My separated material energies.
>
> Besides these, O mighty-armed Arjuna, there is another, superior energy of Mine, which comprises the living entities who are exploiting the resources of this material, inferior nature.
>
> This material nature, which is one of My energies, is working under My direction, O son of Kuntī, producing all moving and nonmoving beings. Under its rule this manifestation is created and annihilated again and again.
>
> It should be understood that all species of life, O son of Kuntī, are made possible by birth in this material nature, and

that I am the seed-giving father.

Sanatan Swami paused and looked over at Kuang Shi, who at that moment was thinking that he had never heard such subject matter expressed so poetically.

"Although an uneducated man may think that it is the mother who gives birth to the child, the wise man knows that it is the father who plants the seed. Similarly, Mother Nature provides the moving and nonmoving beings of the material world— but *only* after being impregnated by the Supreme Father—not independently."

"But you're anthropomorphizing what could just as easily and more convincingly be explained as the result of natural, observable laws," Kuang Shi countered.

"Natural laws do govern the universe and everything in it, but who is the lawmaker?" demanded Sanatan Swami. "The watch has a maker. A baby has a maker. The universe has a maker. Laws don't exist on their own. Who has made them? What is your answer?"

"I know that religion would answer God," retorted Kuang Shi, "but ..."

"... but what does *science* answer?" pressed Sanatan Swami.

Kuang Shi was not going to be easily intimidated. "Science wants proofs! Logic is not a substitute for verifiable investigation," he challenged back.

"But logic is the basis of all good theories," replied the teacher coolly. "Surely you have not forgotten that scientific investigation begins by formulating logical principles. Once this is done, the next step, experimentation, begins. So far, you have been unable to refute the two main principles of *yoga*: A person is a spiritual living entity called the soul, conscious and separate from the body, and there is a supreme intelligent being behind the universe responsible for it. But you have been specifically trained to reject this kind of thinking. Your mind is so much impressed with modern scientific theory that you are willing to accept all of its premises, even though some of them are not at all scientific and have never been proven. You're like a computer, programmed in a set way. As soon as you hear about a supreme intelligent being, you immediately reject the notion as superstition. You have been mis-trained to conclude that the concept of God is nothing more than imagination, when in fact the existence of such a supremely intelligent being is not only logical, but can be proven scientifically. Now if you will simply drop your defenses for a moment and listen with an open mind, I'll describe the process by which that supreme intelligent being can factually be known."

Kuang Shi realized that he was being argumentative, but the topics they were discussing were significant and were of great consequence to him. He was not arguing to prove his own intellectual superiority—he already accepted the Swami's superior intelligence and had no intention of being disrespectful. The conflict was not personal, it was ideological. It was the struggle of two opposing world views of materialism versus spiritualism. And he was fighting on the side of materialism, knowing well that all he had been trained to believe in depended on the outcome. If he failed to defend his convictions, he would not only have to change his way of thinking but even his way of life. He prided himself on being a man of principles living for what he believed in. He would be respectful, but not surrendered. He continued to listen with intense concentration.

"For an experiment to be successful, it must yield predictable results. I intend to prove the existence of the soul within the body as well as the existence of the supremely intelligent being. I'm avoiding the use of the word 'God,' because at present the very word prejudices your thought.

"*Yoga* is the system of proving the existence of the soul

and the supersoul. The word *yoga* means 'link' or 'connection.' By performing *yoga* an individual soul can come to understand his relationship with the supreme soul. Unlike modern scientific researchers, the *yogi* plays dual roles: He is both the researcher as well as the specimen to be studied." "How could anyone remain objective when he himself is the subject of study?" Kuang Shi protested.

"Because there are detailed reference books as well as others practicing *yoga*, he can corroborate his experiments," explained the Swami. "These texts are called the *Vedas*, an encyclopedic body of literature on the science of *yoga*.

"As I mentioned earlier, *yoga* is not just a matter of bodily exercises. That type of *yoga* was especially recommended in ancient times. In each new era, the recommended system of *yoga* changes accordingly. The popular idea of *yoga*—body exercises and breathing techniques—was for a past age. Now it is only useful for maintaining good health."

Kuang Shi again thought of *qigong*. "Have you ever heard of Chinese *qigong*? For what little I know of *yoga*, the two seem to have much in common."

"There are many similarities," acknowledged Sanatan Swami. "Both view the human body as a whole and combine mental, postural, and breathing exercises. I met a number of *qigong* masters during my most recent visit to China, and all of them emphasized the importance of making the mind tranquil and bringing the emotions under control, two important aspects of the *yoga* system."

"My father practices *qigong* every day," Kuang Shi said, "and he rarely gets ill. And as you just mentioned, he is very even-tempered."

"There are many other similarities as well. Both *qigong* and *yoga* recommend regularity in eating, sleeping, work, and recreation," Sanatan Swami added.

"*Qigong* practice is enjoying a new life, thanks to the liberal policies of our government. A recent report I read stated that there are now nearly sixty million followers. There are quite a few research associates also devoted to studying the effects of *qigong* therapy."

"But I suspect that the significance of *qigong* goes beyond the medical benefits. It is over three thousand years old, after all. The *qigong* masters I spoke to described a number of *qigong* schools— Taoist, Buddhist, Confucian, and of course the medical and martial arts schools. The first three saw *qigong* as an intrinsic part of spiritual discipline, where training the body and mind was meant to purify the consciousness. *Yoga* has the very same aim. Though the techniques of *yoga* have changed between ancient times and now, the results achieved from practicing the system of *yoga* in modern times are still the same, purification of one's consciousness. As I was explaining to the audience earlier today, the soul travels from one body to another, and its original pure consciousness becomes covered by material bodily conceptions. This is a contaminated consciousness, and it causes the soul to suffer repeated births and deaths in the material world. Only by purifying the consciousness of all material thoughts and desires can he free himself from yet another material birth. This purified state of consciousness is called Krishna consciousness. In that condition, the soul regains his original spiritual body and enjoys life eternally, full of knowledge and bliss."

"But this is only theory," complained Kuang Shi. "You haven't yet described the actual process, the experiment."

"I was just coming to that," assured the teacher, requesting Kuang Shi's patience. "The actual system of *yoga* recommended for the modern age is known as *bhakti-yoga*, or the science of devotional service to the Supreme Being. According to *yoga*, the individual soul has an eternal relationship with the Supreme Soul. The individual soul is the servant, the Supreme Soul the master. Of course, in the material world no one wants to be anyone's servant, because if you serve someone else, he or she tends to take unfair advantage of you. Thus, everyone wants to be a master and none a servant. Purifying his consciousness by *bhakti-yoga*, the living entity becomes freed of all ignorance and engages once again in the service of the Supreme Soul. But unlike the false masters of this material world, the Supreme Soul is the perfect loving master, and serving Him brings complete satisfaction to the individual soul."

Kuang Shi was growing increasingly impatient. "This is still theory," he complained.

"Don't be so impatient!" Kuang Shi was silenced by Sanatan Swami's reprimand. "You have given twenty years of your life to material education, but you expect to be given spiritual knowledge in less than one hour! Now listen carefully. The aim of the *yoga* experiment is to purify the consciousness. Just as the body is cleansed by bathing with water, to purify the mind and intelligence of contamination a special method of cleansing is required. That method is called *mantra*. *Man* means 'mind,' and *tra* means 'to purify,' or 'to free.' *Mantra* is a sound vibration which purifies the mind. It is the principal step in the *bhakti-yoga* experiment. By hearing repeatedly the spiritual sound vibration of the *mantra*, a person's consciousness becomes purified of all contamination. Here," said Sanatan Swami, handing Kuang Shi a small card on which were written the words:

> Hare Krishna, Hare Krishna
> Krishna Krishna, Hare Hare
> Hare Rama, Hare Rama
> Rama Rama, Hare Hare

Kuang Shi read the card without understanding it. He tried to pronounce the words aloud, like someone reading a foreign language for the first time. Sanatan Swami helped him out.

"Isn't this the same language you were speaking earlier, Sanskrit? What does it mean?"

" 'Krishna' means 'He who is all-attractive,' and 'Rama' means the 'ocean of unlimited pleasure.' Both are names of the Supreme Being. 'Hare' is an address to the energy of the Supreme. The *mantra* is effective because it contains the full unlimited potency of the Supreme, and so by repeating this *mantra* as much as possible, all that is impure in one's mind and heart will be completely cleansed."

"It actually can do that?" asked Kuang Shi.

"Yes!" The confidence with which Sanatan Swami replied dispelled much of Kuang Shi's doubt. "I'll show you how to chant." Sanatan Swami closed his eyes and began:

> Hare Krishna, Hare Krishna
> Krishna Krishna, Hare Hare
> Hare Rama, Hare Rama
> Rama Rama, Hare Hare

Over and over again he repeated the *mantra*, gradually increasing in speed and volume until he became fully absorbed in the sacred prayer. Kuang Shi watched intently, like a scientist observing an experiment. So intense was Sanatan Swami's meditation that Kuang Shi almost expected him to rise off the ground like a mystic *yogi*. Gradually he slowed down his chanting and stopped. Opening his eyes, he looked at Kuang Shi. Kuang Shi sensed a deep inner satisfaction. "How do you feel," he asked almost clinically.

"When I chant Hare Krishna, I feel the greatest happiness. It's like bathing my mind in a shower of nectar. Why don't you try it?"

"Well, I ... ," Kuang Shi stammered, unprepared. "I have to understand a lot more first."

"What kind of scientist are you?" berated the Swami. "When it comes time to perform the experiment, you hesitate. That's the problem with you material scientists—you're ready to experiment on mice and monkeys, but not on yourselves. This science can be fully understood only by *self*-realization. Unless you are willing to perform the experiment personally, you won't understand anything I've been saying. You're the one who's been asking for something besides theory."

Kuang Shi felt embarrassed. It was not that he couldn't chant. He could. In fact he wanted to, but something held him back, as if by chanting he would lose his scientific objectivity.

"If I hand you a bottle of honey and tell you how sweet it tastes, can my words alone convince you? No. You have to taste the honey yourself, and then you'll understand. Just hearing me describe the honey is like licking the outside of the bottle and not tasting the honey itself. Thus far you have heard me describe the philosophy of *yoga*, but you haven't experimented with it. Don't be afraid, I'll help you. Let's chant the *mantra* together." Sanatan Swami pointed to the words on the card and began to chant the *mantra* slowly. His friendly encouragement broke through Kuang Shi's defenses, and he began to chant along:

> Hare Krishna, Hare Krishna
> Krishna Krishna, Hare Hare
> Hare Rama, Hare Rama
> Rama Rama, Hare Hare

Over and over they chanted—so long, in fact, that

Kuang Shi began to look at his watch and wondered when they were going to stop. Sanatan Swami's eyes were closed as he absorbed himself in the sound. No longer hearing Kuang Shi's chanting, he looked to see what was the matter.

"I don't feel anything," said Kuang Shi, as if to explain why he had stopped.

"It takes time," said Sanatan Swami with reassurance. "When one suffers from a chronic disease, even the best medicine requires time before it starts to take effect. Chanting Hare Krishna is the best medicine to cure the disease of chronic materialism. If after taking a bath you are still not clean, you have to bathe again. Similarly, if after chanting the mind is still not purified, it must have been very contaminated and requires further cleansing."

"How *much* cleansing? How much do I have to chant?" interjected Kuang Shi.

"Masters of *yoga* have recommended at least two hours a day of individual chanting as well as further chanting along with others in a group. By regular daily chanting of the Hare Krishna *mantra* you will soon feel relief from all material distress. In other words, no more anxiety."

"But the causes of material distress would still be there," objected Kuang Shi. "I don't want to make believe they're not there!"

"Material existence is not only chronic, it's an epidemic. When there are widespread epidemics such as cholera or flu, the government inoculates all the citizens. The deadly virus is still present, but those who are immunized are safe. In other words, so long as we are in the material world, we cannot eliminate the miseries of material existence, but by chanting Hare Krishna we can at least immunize ourselves and thus avoid the suffering. Only when we become fully Krishna conscious, conscious both of ourselves and our relationship with the Supreme, will we become qualified to leave the diseased world and return to that place which is free from all suffering."

"This kind of experiment could take a very long time," said Kuang Shi hopelessly. He was willing to concede that chanting Hare Krishna might work, but the question was how long until one received the benefits.

"That depends on you. When a patient is given medicine, the doctor also recommends certain other conditions which can speed up the recovery time—for example, taking extra rest. Even in a scientific investigation, there are certain set conditions for the experiment to work. The science of self-realization works the same way. If you want to experience the full benefit of chanting Hare Krishna, you must follow certain regulative principles—no eating of meat, no taking of intoxicants, no gambling, and no illicit sex."

"That's very difficult," Kuang Shi admitted, disconcerted.

"The most worthwhile things are always the most difficult to attain," came Sanatan Swami's reply in a voice firm with the very determination he was trying to encourage Kuang Shi to develop. "Are you afraid of work? I've never known the Chinese people to be lazy. They are perhaps the most industrious people in the world. Now, if only they applied their energy properly, their achievements would be monumental. If they take up the scientific process of *bhakti-yoga*, then by the middle of the twenty-first century they will not only have equalled the other industrialized nations materially, they will have completely surpassed them spiritually. Let future history books record how Krishna consciousness enabled the Chinese people to achieve a level of success in science and culture unique in the modern world!" Sanatan Swami's eyes were ablaze with excitement as he observed the young Chinese man beside him. He was reminded of a similar time many years ago when his own spiritual master had said to him with the same prophetic voice, "Let the history books record how Krishna consciousness saved the world." At the time he also felt a similar disbelief he now saw in the eyes of Kuang Shi. But as time passed, as he saw millions of persons around the world benefited by Krishna consciousness, all his doubts had been removed. "You think it only a dream? Well, ..."

Their attention was suddenly diverted by a rustling sound in the bushes. Struggling with grocery bags, Ananta emerged from the circle of trees into their midst, smiling brightly though a bit out of breath. Both Kuang Shi and Sanatan Swami rose quickly to relieve him.

6

"ANANTA! WHAT TOOK YOU so long?" Sanatan Swami said, relieving his disciple of the weight of the bags.

"It took a while to gather everything. The devotees were still cooking when I got there. I wanted to get a little of each preparation so that Charles—"

"Kuang Shi," corrected the teacher.

"—yes, so that Kuang Shi could experience all the different flavors." Ananta began to spread a large cloth and unpacked the bags. He set a large metal plate and steel cup before his teacher. For Kuang Shi and himself he arranged simple paper plates and cups. He began to name each preparation as he unwrapped them. 'This is a curry of peas, tomatoes, and cheese. The next one is a nice combination of sauteed eggplant and deep-fried potatoes. *Puris*—our bread. Poppers—spicy thin bean wafers. And two types of rice, plain and fancy, cooked with saffron and mixed with cashews and raisins." Reaching into another bag, Ananta added. "This is called *dahl*, a nutritious soup made from beans. I've brought some special delicacies: samosas, which are stuffed vegetable pastries, as well as cauliflower and potato pakoras, which are deep-fried in a chickpea batter. You dip them in this chutney, a coconut sauce." He then moved to the side of his spiritual master to begin serving.

"First serve our guest," Sanatan Swami said. "Oh no, I really couldn't," protested Kuang Shi. Though he had been listening with interest to the menu, he had no intention of eating. "I have to attend a dinner this evening held in my honor. I'm afraid I won't have any appetite if I eat all this."

"Just give him a taste of each," Sanatan Swami instructed his disciple. "A dinner held in your honor?"

"My uncle owns a restaurant in Chinatown, and he's invited all his friends to celebrate my doctorate. Please! Not so much!" Ananta heaped a serving of the peas and curd vegetable on Kuang Shi's plate.

Sanatan Swami chuckled. "There's no need to measure each amount. This is a picnic, not a science lab," he joked. Unable to refuse the hospitality, Kuang Shi nevertheless kept his eye on Ananta.

"Do you eat this much every day?" he asked.

"No," Sanatan Swami laughed. "Today is special. We're celebrating your becoming a doctor." They laughed. The Swami was relaxed, enjoying the rare leisure of an afternoon picnic in the park. His heavy responsibilities and busy schedule did not often afford such an opportunity, and he was savoring every moment. Ananta, too, was especially happy for the chance to serve his spiritual master in such an intimate setting. It was a treasured moment.

"There is a nice story about another doctor, Dr. Frog, who was paid a visit one day by his cousin, who had come from his ocean home. Having never ventured far from his small well. Dr. Frog inquired, 'How big is this ocean you live in? Is it bigger than my well?'

" 'Oh, much bigger!' replied his cousin.

" 'How much bigger?' he asked. 'Twice as big?'

His cousin simply laughed at his limited knowledge.

" 'Well!' he demanded impatiently. 'How much water is there in your ocean!' Straining to comprehend the size of the ocean, he took one deep breath after another, blowing his body to three times his normal size. 'Is it three times bigger than my well?' He puffed again. 'Four times? Five times?' His cousin shook his head. But just as he puffed himself up to six times his usual size, he exploded."

All three now laughed, while Kuang Shi considered the moral.

"Can you guess the meaning?" asked the Swami, still enjoying it. Kuang Shi had a pretty good idea, but chose to be quiet.

"Material scientists are like Dr. Frog. Their attempts to understand the unlimited nature of creation solely in terms of their limited knowledge will bring them to the same end as Dr. Frog."

Though the joke was at his expense, Kuang Shi took it good-naturedly. "Yes, I may be a Dr. Frog. But if my stomach bursts, it will be because you have fed me too much." Again they laughed.

Ananta finished serving his spiritual master and awaited further instructions. "Won't you be joining us?" asked Kuang Shi. He admired Ananta's devotion for his spiritual master. Such reverence did not seem out of place for a person as deserving as Sanatan Swami. Because Kuang Shi himself felt great respect for the elder monk, he appreciated Ananta's behavior.

"No, I'm satisfied just to serve," Ananta replied. "I'll eat later."

"Why don't you eat with us?" said his spiritual master. Ananta began to prepare a plate for himself. The Swami encouraged Kuang Shi to begin eating while everything was still hot. Kuang Shi eyed the variety of foods, uncertain which to try first. He glanced at the teacher. Sanatan Swami was absorbed in relishing the taste of each preparation. His eyes closed, he approached the act of eating with the same meditative mood as when he was chanting. He sat cross-legged, leaning over the plate.

Kuang Shi began to sample each item. The tastes were unusual, but he liked them. They were spicy and a little hot. It reminded him of Szechuan cooking. "It's spicy!"

"Is it too hot for you?" asked the Swami.

"No, my mother uses lots of ginger in her cooking."

"Well, how do you like it?" inquired Ananta, who, by this time had also begun eating.

"It's certainly different from any other food I've eaten, but I like it," Kuang Shi said. He savored each mouthful, relishing the different combinations.

"There's still hope for you, even though you're a scientist," Sanatan Swami joked. "We may still make a *yogi* out of you one day."

"You eat only vegetarian food? How do you get enough protein without meat?"

"There is ample protein in grains like rice, wheat, and corn. Eaten in combination with beans—just like this soup—they are a perfect protein. And there are additional proteins from milk products. You don't have to eat meat, fish, or eggs to be strong. The most powerful animal, the elephant, is a vegetarian. Besides, I could give you many medical arguments in support of a vegetarian diet. But our main reason for avoiding meat, fish, and eggs is that we consider eating an integral part of our *yoga* practice. You would be surprised to know that the cooks never taste anything while cooking. They even try to avoid smelling."

"How is that possible?" Kuang Shi questioned.

"By devotion. We don't cook to please our senses. While cooking, we meditate on the Supreme Lord and when everything is completed, we make an offering to Him.

"*Yoga* is a way of life which incorporates all one's daily activities, and offering everything to the Supreme Lord is the perfection of *yoga*. When the Supreme Lord is fully satisfied with the *yogi*'s offerings, He reveals Himself. This is the final goal of *yoga*, the final proof.

"Seeing the Supreme Lord face to face and entering into a loving relationship with Him, the *yogi* no longer has any doubt about the existence of God, who is seen as a tangible reality. Therefore the experiment involves not only chanting the Hare Krishna *mantra* but includes all activities performed as service to the Supreme Lord.

"An example is cooking. Though the Lord lacks nothing, being the source of the entire creation, He nevertheless accepts food when it is prepared and offered to Him with love. Whatever is accepted by the Lord becomes transformed into spiritual energy, and we call such food prasadam, which means 'the mercy of the Lord.' Eating such sanctified food purifies our consciousness."

Kuang Shi had been following the teacher's explanation carefully. But the idea of something material becoming spiritual did not seem at all scientific. "I cannot understand how this food which we are eating is different from any other food, except of course for the difference in spicing. Just how does matter become anti-matter?"

Sanatan Swami ate the last part of a vegetable-filled pastry. "There is a practical example which may help to clear up the point. In ironworking, large pieces of metal are often reshaped by bending them under very high temperature. Although iron is a metal, when it is put in the fire it becomes red-hot and takes on all the qualities of the fire itself. It is more like fire than iron. In the same way, whatever is offered to the Supreme Lord loses its material nature and instead takes on the spiritual qualities of the

Lord. In the ancient teachings there are examples of persons who became purified simply by eating sanctified food which had been offered to the Lord. As the ancient Vedic teachings are free of any mistakes, we must accept such testimony as reliable evidence, just as we would accept the records of any trustworthy scientist."

Ananta had been following the conversation and added, "You may think this food ordinary, but you will start to feel the effects soon enough."

"Now he probably thinks you've put some drug into the food and he won't eat any more," joked the master.

Kuang Shi's ever-quizzical mind had thought of another question. "If food becomes spiritualized by being offered to God, why not offer Him meat?"

This question pleased Sanatan Swami. He stopped eating and paused for a moment. "If we accept the premise that the purpose of *yoga* is to please the Supreme, then shouldn't we find out what pleases Him most before offering Him anything? The *Bhagavad-gītā* advises:

> If one offers Me with love and devotion a leaf, a flower, fruit or water, I will accept it.

"It is clear from this statement that the Supreme Lord does not accept offerings which include meat, fish, and eggs, and this is why we do not eat these things. If He accepted them, then we would certainly offer them. But since they can't be offered, we would be eating lumps of sin in the form of dead flesh. This is also described in the *Bhagavad-gītā*:

> The devotees of the Lord are released from all kinds of sin because they eat food which is offered first for sacrifice. Others, who prepare food for personal sense enjoyment, verily eat only sin.

Yoga for the New Millennium

"Okay, but what I want to know is what exactly do you mean by 'sin'?" Kuang Shi asked.

"Now we're getting to the real issue, and the point is this: Any activity performed against the recommendation of Vedic literature is called a sin. Now," he added for emphasis, "we're talking about issues which touch our very lives. I know you've been listening carefully, but please pay special attention. We are all eternal servants of the Supreme Lord, but we forget this essential truth and instead become lost in selfish activities, which are the very basis of sin. Our suffering, therefore, is caused by sinful activities performed both in this life as well as past lifetimes. Material nature, working under the direction of the Supreme Lord, awards the results for all our actions, both good and bad. The living entity thus enjoys or suffers according to his own deeds. The *Bhagavad-gītā* clearly states this:

> Nature is said to be the cause of all material causes and effects, whereas the living entity is the cause of the various sufferings and enjoyments in this world.
>
> The living entity in material nature thus follows the ways of life, enjoying the three modes of nature. This is due to his association with that material nature. Thus he meets with good and evil amongst various species.

"You mean I was born in a crowded country like China because of what I might have done in a past life?" Kuang Shi was grasping for a clear understanding.

"Exactly! Like your billion or so countrymen, you've taken birth in China because of reactions to your past deeds. Overpopulation or not, it's the principle of what you have done in lifetimes past that has determined your birth in that particular country. Some people are born in deserts, others in teeming cities like Shanghai or Tokyo. The very same law of nature determines the birth of every living entity and his transmigration throughout the numerous species of life. The number of actual spiritual beings remains the same throughout creation. Where they transmigrate from one lifetime to another depends on what they have done—or not done—in the past.

"Just as in physics a particular action yields a predictable reaction, this scientific knowledge in the *Vedas* describes the law of *karma*, or the law of action and reaction. Just as the government rewards its faithful citizens while punishing law-breakers, the Supreme Lord, who is the ultimate judge, awards or punishes each person according to his actions. There is no such thing as 'luck.' "

Kuang Shi interrupted, "I beg your pardon, but I'll have to differ with you on this point. Heisenberg has conclusively proven that uncertainty, or chance—or perhaps as you would have it, luck—is one of the fundamental principles governing all universal activity, including the smallest particles of creation."

Sanatan Swami immediately countered, "Yes, but what he failed to acknowledge was the far more fundamental principle of cause and effect. Every effect has a past cause. Fair enough?" Kuang Shi nodded. "Then who or what caused the principle of uncertainty? We see that someone who works very hard may not always become wealthy, but someone else with only a slight endeavor becomes very rich. It sounds like chance, but actually the unseen factor is the hand of God awarding the results of past lives' activities. In the same way someone may be born with a defect at birth— perhaps blindness. Are you going to tell me that this was due to 'uncertainty' or bad luck? No. This is the result of some past sinful activity."

Kuang Shi fell silent. After a long pause, he cleared his throat and said, "What would be the result, for example, of my eating meat or fish?"

"Well, according to the *Vedas*, one who kills another living entity or even causes it to be killed for his own selfish needs, has to suffer the same reaction in a future life."

"Do you mean to say that if I eat steak or chicken tonight, I will be born as a cow or a chicken only to be slaughtered? I don't believe it."

"Believe or not believe, the law of karma will act. Are you willing to take the risk of being slaughtered just to satisfy the momentary desires of your tongue?" Sanatan Swami asked soberly.

"But if I don't know any better—if I don't know the law of karma—then why should I have to suffer?" protested Kuang Shi.

"Ignorance is no excuse. Due to ignorance, a child may put his hand in the fire, but will that stop the child from getting burned?"

"Well, it doesn't seem fair to me," said Kuang Shi. "Why should I be held responsible for everything that happens to me?" All this was making him feel uneasy and he lost interest in the meal.

Smiling, Sanatan Swami tried to console him. "After all, it was our choice that we left the spiritual world to come here in the first place, and it is also our choice how long we wish to stay here. Those who are intelligent take advantage of this spiritual knowledge and avoid committing further sins. The *Bhagavad-gītā* states:

> Persons who have acted piously in previous lives and in this life and whose sinful actions are completely eradicated are freed from the dualities of delusion, and they engage themselves in My service with determination.

"Thus their lives become virtually free from suffering, and in the end they return to the spiritual world, no longer to suffer the repetition of birth and death. These are perfect *yogis*."

"I still can't see why ignorance is punished. Isn't education preferable?"

"Education is always preferable," agreed Sanatan Swami, "but it is not always possible. Some people refuse to be educated. Don't all governments maintain strict discipline for those who break the law? The government tries its best to educate everyone, but when all else fails it has no alternative but to resort to punishment. If people insist on ignoring scriptural guidelines like the *Bhagavad-gītā*, what alternative is there for God?"

"But a criminal knows when he's breaking the law. He deserves to be punished. But most people have never heard of the law of karma. Why should they be punished?" The law of karma just didn't sit well with Kuang Shi. He felt he wanted to make a move toward spiritual life but felt himself held back. He couldn't immediately loosen himself from everything he had been—his culture, his education, his conditioning, his background, his beliefs. It all seemed so difficult. But Sanatan Swami cut through it all.

"If you feel so concerned, why don't you devote your life to learning and teaching this science? That's what I've done. In more than twenty years I've never asked for any payment nor taken a single day off for a vacation. I'm dedicated to freeing people from ignorance."

"I'm also trying to do that in my own way," was Kuang Shi's response.

The Swami was not impressed. "You haven't understood what I've been saying about the law of karma. You see, ultimately it is benevolent, much in the same way that a prison is ideally meant to correct the lawbreaker, not simply to punish him. You can't blame the government for building a prison. It's the only way to protect innocent citizens from the criminals. Even within the confinement of the prison, the state is always making efforts to educate them. And if a prisoner sincerely repents, he's sometimes released before his sentence expires.

"In the same way, we're all convicts in the prison house of this material world. Through the commission of so many sinful activities, under the law of *karma* each one of us has been sentenced to serve in the prison of a material body. If we realize our mistake and abide by God's laws, we can gain our freedom from the material world and return to our original place as eternal servants of the Supreme Lord. The alternative is simply more sinful activities and therefore repeated imprisonment. The choice is ours. Do you really want to help your fellow man?"

"Yes, certainly," replied Kuang Shi. "Especially in places like China, which are technologically backward."

"If you really want to serve your people, then teach them to be Krishna conscious. No doubt China can be improved by scientific advancement, but the material miseries of life will continue."

"But even temporary relief is some help. At least one can then look for a final solution. First you feed a starving man, then teach him how to work," said Kuang Shi pragmatically.

"Many welfare workers are already offering temporary relief," said Sanatan Swami, "but they're unable to free anyone from the chains of sinful reactions. They're like the blind leading the blind. Your father gave you the name 'Kuang Shi,' and there can be no greater charity than to teach Krishna consciousness. How long have you been in America?"

"Nearly five years," responded Kuang Shi.

"For five years you've been on the receiving end. Don't you think it's about time to be giving in return? What I'm suggesting is that you not only fulfill the hopes of your government, not only live up to the great name your father gave you, but that you surpass all their expectations. Teach the Chinese people that their true destiny is not only to achieve the status of a developed nation by the middle of the twenty-first century, but that the highest achievement of human existence is spiritual; an eternal life full of knowledge and perfect happiness. In this way you will bring glory to your nation and to the entire world."

Kuang Shi was speechless.

"We've been here more than an hour," Sanatan Swami said, looking at his watch. As he stood up, adjusting his saffron robe, Kuang Shi sat thoughtfully. With his incisive vision, Sanatan Swami had just revealed that if, after his five long years of effort to gain a Ph.D., he continued to ignore his duty to his nation and his people, he was really no better than a miser. Facing the spiritual master and his disciple, Kuang Shi felt decidedly vulnerable. The surrounding trees were like a silent tribunal waiting for his decision, the overhead sun affording no shadow to hide within. The two devotees who for the last hour had shown him such personal attention were now busy packing their bags, leaving him with only his thoughts. He stumbled for words.

"I ... where are you going?" he managed to ask.

"We have to get back to our Festival of India. There must be thousands of persons there by now," explained Ananta.

"Of course we give special attention to thoughtful, educated people like yourself," said Sanatan Swami. "But intellectuals are quite common these days, especially in New York City. Now, if we were to meet a representative of China's more than one billion people, that would certainly warrant our complete, undivided attention." The Swami's mild irony brought a smile to Kuang Shi's face. "We're not quite certain whom we're dealing with, a future scientist or a future reformer."

"Perhaps both," was Kuang Shi's quick response.

"Then we shall have to treat you accordingly. Mr.

Scientist, may we present you with this scientific treatise of spiritual knowledge—the *Bhagavad-gītā*—containing elaborate knowledge, noumenal and phenomenal. Mr. Reformer, please accept this gift—the *Bhagavad-gītā*—a directive for the spiritual upliftment of mankind."

Kuang Shi accepted the gift graciously. From his previous night's reading and while listening to the master's discourse, the *Bhagavad-gītā*'s authority had been repeatedly cited. Now he would have an opportunity to study it firsthand. He was filled with excitement at the thought of delving into this treasure-house of knowledge.

"What are you doing tomorrow?" Ananta's question drew Kuang Shi's attention.

"I'm afraid I'm going to be busy at my relatives."

"Oh, that's too bad." Ananta added, "because I wanted to invite you to our cultural center."

Kuang Shi thought for a moment and then replied, "Perhaps you can come to my university some time next week. I'd really like you to meet some of my friends. I'm sure they'd have many intelligent questions."

"Which university?" Sanatan Swami asked.

"Columbia."

"I think you're free Tuesday evening," Ananta said, looking at his spiritual master.

"I'd love to come," Sanatan Swami responded. Kuang Shi wrote down his dormitory address and gave it to Ananta.

"Would 7:00 p.m. be alright?"

Sanatan Swami was visibly pleased. "Fine. We meet Tuesday. Ananta, give Kuang Shi a few small books to give to his friends. I've very much enjoyed our discussion today. I think our meeting has been arranged by Krishna."

"Yes," agreed Kuang Shi, "I think so too." And as he followed the spiritual teacher and his assistant out of the circle of trees and through the bushes, retracing their path to the side of the lake, Kuang Shi had the distinct feeling that there must certainly be some supernatural force at work. Krishna?

7

"A TOAST! A TOAST!"

"Yes, let's have a toast!" echoed a voice from a nearby table. Lawrence Chung stood proudly, a wine glass held high in one hand, while with the other he gripped the back of his chair to steady himself. Again he attempted to make himself heard above the din of the nearly two hundred guests who had come in response to his invitation. As one course followed another and wine glasses were filled and refilled, spirits ran high. Waiters bustled about, clearing the tables, while others rushed through the stairway doors with yet more platters. The air was thick with cigarette smoke hovering like clouds over each table. The tinkling of dinnerware merged with conversations and Chinese music to create a cacophony of sound. But no one seemed to notice, much less mind. Rather, it heightened the festive party mood.

Lawrence Chung's round, bald face gave no indication of any frustration for not being heard. He had been drinking from early evening and was feeling pleasantly drunk. His usual pale complexion was suffused with a redness which spread out from his nose in all directions due to the warming effect of the wine he had been consuming. His tie was pulled much too tightly against the stiff shirt collar framing his customary dark blue suit, creating the uncomfortable impression of one suffering from strangulation. He was tapping his glass with a soup spoon, trying vainly to attract attention.

"Chung Shi Long, please sit down!" urged Shiao Lin,

pulling on her husband's jacket. She did not expect him to obey but felt compelled to make a show of propriety for her best friend, Yang Po Ling, who sat to her left. Observing her husband's indifference, she leaned in front of him and addressed Kuang Shi. "You have not even touched the roast pork. Is something wrong? I promised your mother I would look after you just like my own son, so do not disappoint me. Eat nicely."

"Dear Auntie, I'm stuffed to my neck already. I cannot eat another bite." He was not being untruthful. Uncle Lawrence had given the order to serve every dish on the menu, and as the guest of honor Kuang Shi had felt obliged to try each one. At the present moment, he felt as stuffed as the roast pig which the waiters were wheeling on a cart from table to table, carving slices for each guest. Seeing the roasted animal being carted about, its eyes fixed in a glassy stare and a burnt apple propping open its mouth, he realized suddenly that a day or so ago it had probably been alive and breathing as much as anyone in the room. The lessons of the early afternoon, the message of the *Bhagavad-gītā*, seemed to call out: within this animal there had been a soul, a living soul like anyone else. Now that soul was gone, leaving only a fleshy corpse. And there was a still more disturbing lesson, wasn't there? Those who sat feasting upon this flesh would themselves be feasted upon in some future birth. It was mortifying. Kuang Shi refused the slice of pork on the plea of having already overeaten. He didn't mention his real reason.

Kuang Shi felt the elbow of Jimmy Allen, his uncle's best friend and golfing partner, nudging him. "It looks like your uncle could use a bit of help," rumbled the real-estate broker. Rising to his host's side, Jimmy Allen's 6-foot 4-inch, 240-pound body dwarfed Kuang Shi's uncle. "Ladies and gentlemen! Ladies and gentlemen!" he bellowed loudly. "May I have your attention!" His powerful voice brought the room to a hushed silence. "Larry's trying to make a speech, so let's hear him." He turned to Larry and then sat down, having accomplished his task.

"Thank you, Jimmy," he acknowledged gratefully. "And thanks to all of you for coming here this evening to honor my nephew Charlie Li." He pulled his somewhat embarrassed nephew to his side and placed his arm around his shoulder in familial affection. "Soon to be Doctor Charles Li." There was a loud burst of applause and cheers from all the tables. The host quieted his guests with a wave of his arm.

He surveyed the banquet room's fifteen linen-covered tables around which sat his friends, relatives, business associates, important acquaintances, and leading citizens of Chinatown, all accompanied by their wives. They were the familiar faces of all his well-wishers, come to celebrate his family's good fortune. Seeing their happy faces made him flushed with pride.

"Many of us sitting here tonight know how this boy must be feeling. Many of us also came with nothing but holes in our pockets." There was a burst of appreciative laughter. "Now those hard times are behind us and we laugh remembering them. Seeing this young man standing before us calls for a toast, a toast to his achievement and also to this great nation, the United States of America." While wine glasses clinked, cries of "America!" "Free enterprise!" "Charlie!" rent the air. Again the host quieted his ebullient guests with a wave. "I wish Kuang Shi's parents were here tonight to share this moment with us. Every father and mother should be so fortunate to have a child who can fulfill their dreams. After all, our hard work is meant for them."

From a distant table: "A toast to the kids! Our future hope!"

"I started as a dishwasher at the China Dragon. Those

times were so tough I sometimes wondered if I had made a mistake in coming here." Under the influence of wine, amidst so many friends, Larry Chung was becoming emotional. He rested his hand on his wife's shoulder, tears welling in his eyes as he scanned the faces of his many friends. "Without your support. I'd still be washing dishes."

"We're still with you, Larry!" said a voice from a nearby table, with others similarly affirming.

"You're the greatest friends a man could have," said Larry deeply moved. "All I can say is thank you. Thank you for everything." Seeing their host choked with emotion and unable to speak further, they returned their appreciation with loud applause, to which Larry waved, sitting down, quite overwhelmed.

"You're a lucky man to have an uncle like Larry," said Jimmy Allen, as Kuang Shi settled back into his seat between Mr. Allen and his uncle. "There aren't many men who can gather this many friends on only twenty-four hours' notice."

"What to speak of making such first-class arrangements!" added Arnold Rosen, owner of the next-door jewelry shop and Larry's neighbor and friend for the past twenty years. His square, black-framed spectacles, thick black hair and bushy eyebrows gave Arnold, thin and in his late fifties, an especially penetrating appearance. In contrast, his rotund wife Sally, sitting between her husband and Jimmy Allen, radiated frivolity with her bleached blond hair, heavy makeup, and excited laughter, which she released at the slightest provocation. At the moment she was navigating her way through the "Dragon Soup," a specialty of the restaurant, examining the mysterious ingredients in her spoon before consuming them.

Noticing Mrs. Rosen's hesitation, Jimmy Allen reassured her that she was indeed treading in safe waters. "The Chinese eat everything that flies except kites, anything with legs except chairs, and anything that swims except a boat," he joked in a hushed voice still loud enough to be heard by everyone else at the table. This sent Mrs. Rosen into a fit of giggles, despite her husband Arnold's disdainful looks.

From across the table, Mr. Fang Ming Wai, president of the Chinatown Merchants Association, objected, "That's not at all true, Mr. Allen. On the contrary, we Chinese are very fond of kites and chairs." Plump Mrs. Rosen's double chin shook with delight as laughter quickly enveloped everyone, because the remark had come from a usually serious Chinese elderman.

Embarrassed by his wife's tittering, Arnold Rosen sought to divert the others' attention by raising a more political subject. Though a businessman by profession, he prided himself for having received a university degree in history and kept abreast of current world affairs. Addressing Mr. Fang with noticeable solemnity, he said, "I'm a little disappointed with the direction China is taking these days. What has happened to the idealism of the earlier years immediately following Liberation? When I read about some of the reforms now being instituted it sounds more like pure capitalism rather than social reform."

"I'm surprised to hear such remarks from an American businessman," replied Mr. Fang coolly. "Every Chinese man and woman I know feels nothing but relief at the turn of events. And that goes for Chinese in China as well as overseas. There's nothing wrong with profit-making if it's achieved legitimately," Mr. Fang said, expertly pouring himself a cup of tea. Having done business in Chinatown for so many years Arnold Rosen had developed respect for elders like Fang Ming Wai, and so he decided not to offer any more argument.

Kuang Shi had been listening with only mild interest, Looking around the room at the others, he was struck by the contrast between them and the personality of Sanatan Swami. He recalled the sublime meeting with the spiritual master earlier in the day. In comparison with this hot and smoky room, the cool, fresh atmosphere of the park seemed so attractive. After their meeting, Kuang Shi had spent nearly two hours reading *Bhagavad-gītā* and now happily noticed his own disinterest in all the table talk. He found himself much preferring the gravity and wisdom of Sanatan Swami.

Kuang Shi also thought about Ananta, who, though still young, was quite mature and already appeared to understand life's ultimate purpose. Kuang Shi looked to his aunt, her friend Yang Po Ling, Mrs. Yang's daughter Carolyn, and to his young cousins Johnny and Susan, who were listening with small earphones to a Sony Walkman. Both were smiling, happy in their teenage world and utterly indifferent to what was going on at the table. In fact, Kuang Shi thought, they looked rather out of place dressed in such formal clothes. He was accustomed to seeing Johnny in his shorts, T-shirt, and sneakers bouncing a basketball down the street, Susan riding her bicycle with her friends. Kuang Shi laughed at his realization that they were nearly the same age as Ananta yet lifetimes apart.

He looked to Susan's right. Carolyn Yang had been staring at him and their eyes now met. She was a sophomore at New York University. Ever since Kuang Shi had come to America, Carolyn's mother had been eyeing him as a possible husband for her daughter. Mr. Yang had passed away more than ten years earlier, leaving substantial wealth to his wife and daughter. The energetic Mrs. Yang had increased their savings, so they were under no financial pressures. Marrying her daughter to a Ph.D. would add prestige to the wealth they already had. The advantages would be mutual, Po Ling often emphasized to her friend Shiao Lin. When the young man's studies were completed he would no longer be able to stay in America on his student visa. Carolyn was a U.S. citizen having been born here. If Charles were to marry her, he could easily become a citizen as well.

Kuang Shi was not worried about his visa status. He knew that graduate students of his caliber were always given permanent residency if they wished to stay. He was not very eager to be tied down by marriage, at least for the next few years.

He strained to hear what Mrs. Yang was saying to his aunt. The two were having quite an animated discussion. Kuang Shi heard his aunt mention the name of some of the large corporations which had been anxiously pursuing him with job offers. He watched Mrs. Yang arch her eyebrows when she heard that one company had offered one hundred thousand dollars as a starting salary. She darted a glance at Kuang Shi and, noticing that he had been looking at her, smiled in such a way which made Kuang Shi think that she was hearing wedding bells.

A group of Chinese elders and their wives had come over to the table, and Lawrence Chung stood to thank them for coming. Kuang Shi also stood as each offered congratulations. After they departed, Kuang Shi sat down and looked at his watch. It was past eleven. He looked out across the large banquet hall. Most of the guests were still chatting and leisurely sipping drinks. It was going to be a late night. He would have to wait for all the guests to leave, because everyone would come over and personally extend their best wishes. Kuang Shi closed his eyes. It had been a long day.

8

KUANG SHI MANEUVERED the vacuum cleaner around the leg of the chair, careful to maintain a forward sweeping motion so that the entire rug had a manicured appearance. Satisfied, he flicked the switch, halting the machine's disturbing whine. Silence. He flopped down in the chair and made sure that everything was neat and clean. The late afternoon sun pouring through the window created a stripe across his desk and the dark blue rug. His guests would be arriving momentarily, and he was excited. After all, he rarely entertained visitors in his dormitory room. He was always too busy with his studies. Sometimes an occasional school friend, but never anyone like Sanatan Swami. For a moment he thought he heard them coming—but whoever they were passed by his room, their voices trailing off in the hallway.

He decided to give Winston a call.

"Winston? I'm glad you're there. Have you spoken with David and Ann?" Winston's deep and jovial voice immediately put Kuang Shi at ease.

"Charles, when I promise you I'll do something, do I ever let you down? They've confirmed that they're coming. The others had appointments or just weren't interested. But, listen—you'll never guess who wants to come." Kuang Shi had no idea.

"Come on, guess who!"

"I can't, Winston. Just tell me." Kuang Shi was impatient.

"Red Simon!"

"Red? I don't believe it." Kuang Shi had mixed feelings as he thought of Red Simon. Red was intelligent and fun to be with, but he had the peculiar habit of joking about almost everything. He had purposely avoided telling him about Sanatan Swami's visit, fearing that if he came he might say something that would offend the respected teacher.

"Red was the most eager of all those I spoke to. He's already read some of the Krishna books. He said he's even gone to some of their meetings."

"Well, I just hope he controls himself and doesn't say anything insulting. Carlos is also coming. I guess it'll be an intimate group. I reserved the guest lounge."

There was a knock at the door. "Winston, I think they're here. See you at seven-thirty. Bye." Kuang Shi put the phone down and opened the door.

The smiling faces of Sanatan Swami and Ananta greeted him. "Hare Krishna!" they said together.

"Please come in! I'm so pleased that you've come." Kuang Shi suddenly realized just how pleased he really was. He felt genuinely happy to have their friendly association again. "Please sit here," he said, gesturing to the two easy chairs which occupied the right side of the small room.

Sanatan Swami walked to the desk and looked out at the courtyard park. Turning, he glanced around the room and then seated himself comfortably in the armchair nearest the desk, while Ananta occupied one near the door.

"I would imagine this is quite an improvement over Beijing University?" he said half-jokingly.

"It's much better than anything China can offer," replied Kuang Shi, swiveling his desk chair in their direction. "I would have been embarrassed to invite you there."

"Ananta takes everything for granted. But even I was shocked to see the student living conditions in China."

"You actually visited a dormitory there?" Kuang Shi found it hard to envision the dignified spiritual master in a crowded Beijing students' quarters.

"Yes," Sanatan Swami replied. "I like to observe how people live. It tells you a great deal about them, sometimes more than they will openly admit. For instance, I can guess that it would be very difficult for you to return to your previous way of life, having enjoyed the privacy of this room."

Kuang Shi smiled.

"In the dormitory I visited, there were eight students living in a room no bigger than this. Their clothes were scattered everywhere due to there being so little space to store them. There's no peace of mind in the dormitory." explained Sanatan Swami in answer to Ananta's quizzical look.

"The graduate facilities are slightly better," said Kuang Shi. "Of course, nothing like this."

"The most surprising thing is the lack of proper bathing arrangements. There are no showers."

"No showers?" repeated Ananta with some disbelief. He looked to Kuang Shi for an explanation.

"There are showers but in a separate building." "In the university I visited, the bath house was open only during the class hours. The students I spoke to told me they bathe only once a week."

"There's a definite need for more hygienic training," admitted Kuang Shi. "But if the facilities existed, I'm sure the students would bathe daily."

"In any case, I think it will be difficult for you to readjust," said the Swami. "Did you get an opportunity to study the *Bhagavad-gītā*?" he asked, changing the subject.

"I spent most of Sunday reading it, and I've got lots of questions. But what I've read has impressed me." The two devotees were happy to hear this.

"And your friends?" asked Ananta. "Did you distribute the books to them?"

"To those I thought might be interested. Anyway, I've been trying to organize this meeting; I'm afraid it was very short notice."

"How many are coming?" asked Ananta.

"Five or six," said Kuang Shi apologetically. "But they're keen to come."

"My spiritual master was willing to speak to an empty room," said Sanatan Swami determinedly. "He often said he was prepared to spend his entire life teaching anyone who sincerely wanted to learn the science of Krishna consciousness. 'Better one moon than many stars,' he would say. At least you'll be present and I've noticed that you listen very attentively, so our time will not be wasted."

Kuang Shi felt honored by the master's confidence in him, though he felt he had done little to warrant it. "It's time to go," he said.

As they rose to leave for the guest reception, Sanatan Swami paused, looking with great earnestness at Kuang Shi: "One who receives this knowledge bears a great responsibility. I'm not speaking simply for your sake. I am thinking of your Chinese brothers and sisters. Do you understand?"

Their eyes met. There was only silence. But in that silence Kuang Shi thought that he heard a pearl drop into a vast and fathomless ocean, a wondrous jewel sounding deep within his heart and echoing off in millions more.

In the reception room on the ground floor, Kuang Shi's friends had already assembled and were waiting for him to arrive with his guests. Carlos sat reading a newspaper, while Red played with a television remote control, randomly changing channels. David and his girlfriend Ann sat on a sofa talking quietly together, as large, heavy-set Winston paced back and forth. Kuang Shi entered, smiling broadly at the others, then turned to introduce Sanatan Swami, who along with Ananta now stood in the center of the room.

"I would like to introduce everyone," he said with formality. "This is Sanatan Swami and Ananta, one of his students." "My name is Winston," said the thick-bearded philosophy graduate from Wisconsin, introducing himself with a friendly handshake. Following Winston's lead, each of the others came forward in turn.

"Please sit here, Maharaj," said Winston with a sweep of his arm, ushering their distinguished guest to the vacant sofa. Kuang Shi figured that the title "Maharaj" probably indicated great respect for a holy person in India. Winston was his best friend, and Kuang Shi appreciated his friend's effort to make the guests feel at home. He hoped that the others would also emulate Winston's respectful mood.

They took their seats, Ananta and Kuang Shi on either side of Sanatan Swami, seated on a large sofa which occupied the entire rear wall, Carlos to their immediate left, with Red beside him. To Ananta's right, beneath the curtained windows, sat Winston, while David and Ann sat on the sofa beside him.

"Perhaps I may briefly introduce each of my friends to you," said Kuang Shi. "Carlos is from Nicaragua. He's a political science major." Everyone, including Carlos, laughed, considering that Nicaragua was embroiled in political turmoil both internally and with the United States.

"Which side are you on?" asked Sanatan Swami.

"I prefer to keep that a secret," Carlos responded with equally good humor. "That way everyone remains my friend."

"Spoken like a true diplomat," Winston quipped.

"And I'm his public relations man. I write all his speeches."

"Winston's a philosophy major," explained Kuang Shi, smiling.

"Yes. When I failed science, math, and all other practical subjects, my professors advised me to try philosophy. It worked. Now everyone considers me a true intellectual."

"That's not true," quipped Red merrily. "It's only since you grew that beard that you actually became wise."

"Winston is right," remarked Sanatan Swami somewhat soberly. "The greatest geniuses often display traits of eccentricity."

"That's certainly true in Winston's case," Red playfully taunted.

Kuang Shi was glad that the meeting had gotten off to a buoyant start and that everyone seemed quite relaxed. But he didn't want it to be so casual that his friends would lose regard for their esteemed guest. Reading the *Bhagavad-gītā* had increased his respect for the spiritual tradition that Sanatan Swami represented. Besides, it was customary for Chinese to honor elders, something that Americans were not in the habit of doing. With noticeable gravity he introduced the others.

"David is a graduate in engineering. His father owns one of the largest construction companies in New York, and this fall he'll be starting to work with his father."

"Actually I've already started. It's a pleasure to meet you," David said politely. He was tall, slim, and blond-haired, with a thin mustache that neatly lined his upper lip. Always well-dressed, he gave the appearance of one destined for success. Ann, his girlfriend since their high school days, was a handsome woman. Her long black hair was pulled back and knotted in a bun. In contrast to David's mild nature, she was strong and outspoken. Kuang Shi respected Ann as a serious, intelligent fellow researcher.

"Ann is specializing in the field of medical research. We've been in many classes together."

"A fellow scientist," appreciated Sanatan Swami.

"And finally, Red Simon," said Kuang Shi. "He's a graduate of the school of business administration." Red's natural bright-orange hair, coupled with his normally frenetic disposition, created mirth wherever he went. Yet he was intelligent and, when necessary, shrewd to the point of cunning.

This was the group that Sanatan Swami now studied. Each had received one or more small books from Kuang Shi, and they were obviously more intelligent than the average person. He decided it would be best not to give a formal lecture since the mood was already light and the group small. Better, Sanatan Swami thought, to engage them in dialogue on topics of interest to them.

Carlos raised the first question. "Charles gave us some of your literature. Frankly, I think these teachings are no longer very relevant to our modern world. For example, in the book I read monarchy is considered the ideal form of government, the king the ideal leader. But doesn't history show us that when authority is reposed in the hands of a single person, or even a select few, authority becomes oppressive and corrupt? Whether by constitutional arrangement or through forceful revolution, nearly every nation has at least theoretically adopted a more representative form of government. As the saying goes, 'Absolute power corrupts absolutely,'" Carlos concluded brusquely and reclined back in his seat.

Sanatan Swami was unfazed by the political rhetoric. "The real issue is that the leadership must always be ideal, regardless of the particular form of government that it takes. Do you really believe that placing power in the hands of many eliminates corruption?"

Kuang Shi considered the situation in China, where the government was instituting major legislation to curb widespread corruption and bribery. And the problem was not limited to China. In the United States the resignation of leading government figures was common. Embarrassing scandals had even claimed a former President.

"In most countries people no longer have faith in their leaders," continued Sanatan Swami. "The *Bhagavad-gītā* states:

> *yad yadācarati śreṣṭhas*
> *tat tad evetaro janaḥ*
> *sa yat pramāṇaṁ kurute*
> *lokas tad anuvartate*

Whatever action a great man performs, common men follow. And whatever standards he sets by exemplary acts, all the world pursues.

"In other words, if the leaders are addicted to bad habits, how can the citizenry behave properly in any way at all? Therefore, what really constitutes moral and ethical behavior is revealed in transcendental literatures like the *Bhagavad-gītā*. A leader's teaching as well as his behavior should be based upon authorized books of knowledge. The heads of the government, the father, and the school teacher are natural authorities for the innocent public and have a great responsibility to their dependents."

"But they are just as susceptible to human frailties as any common man," observed Winston.

"Then they are not truly good leaders," the Swami declared. "One who is a true devotee of God has the highest qualifications in whatever field he chooses to work in. The *Bhagavad-gītā* describes the qualities of just such an ideal person:

One who is not envious but a kind friend to all living entities, who does not think of himself a proprietor, who is free from false ego and equal both in happiness and distress, who is always satisfied and engaged in devotional service with determination and whose mind and intelligence are in agreement with Me—he is very dear to Me.

Yoga for the New Millennium 83

Ann leaned forward, "Your philosophy seems to give more importance to men."

"No, it gives equal importance to all. Our principle is to emphasize the importance of the soul, which is superior to dualities like male and female—not the body."

Kuang Shi studied Ann's reaction. He knew that she would pursue the point further.

"Charles gave me a book in which nearly all the examples cited were that of men. From what little I know of Asian cultures, women are always consigned to subordinate roles. Burdened with rearing many children, they're forced to stay at home without the chance to pursue a career which will contribute to society, something that men take for granted."

"Not all Asian countries are the same," corrected Kuang Shi. "Chinese women are becoming prominent in many fields. Of course it was not always like that, but traditional ideas are slowly giving way to a more scientific understanding of equality between the sexes."

"Scientifically they are not equal. When you get married can you make your husband pregnant?" asked Sanatan Swami pointedly. "There are physiological differences. Equality cannot be found anywhere in nature. No two individuals are alike, and the general rule holds that the weak are subsistence for the strong. It will be impossible for you to establish material equality."

David felt that Ann had been misunderstood. Though usually quiet he now spoke up. "What Ann meant was that everyone should have equal opportunity to..."

"To do what?" interrupted the teacher. "To grow old? To die? For these there are equal opportunities."

David was a bit miffed. "No, the opportunity to realize one's full potential."

"That's not totally within an individual's control. When you go to work for your father, will you be starting at the same level as the others? If you're going to argue for material equality, then the fact that your father owns the business should have no bearing on whether you get the job or how much salary you receive. The fact is, inequality begins at birth."

Kuang Shi studied the faces of the others in the room. Sanatan Swami's ideas were not consistent with popular trends. The atmosphere had become somewhat tense.

Carlos erupted, "I have heard this argument too many times! It has been used for centuries to keep people subjugated."

"You haven't understood," Ananta said. He knew that his spiritual master often stimulated discussion by creating confrontation.

"What the Swami is talking about," Red Simon offered, "is the law of karma. Your birth is determined by the actions of your previous life. Karma explains why you were born in Nicaragua, Charles in China, and all the rest of us in America."

"It also determines why each of us is born with specific qualities," added Ananta.

"You mean genes?" asked Ann.

"Call it by whatever name you will, but the fact is that we're all different. No two peas in the pod are the same."

"But one thing everyone does have in common," Sanatan Swami put in, "which is their primal motivation to improve their lot. The history of the world is nothing if not man's attempt to improve his situation. Yet whatever he achieves is short-lived, for the inexorable forces of material nature will not allow him to enjoy success for very long."

"I just can't agree with you," said Ann. "Mankind is definitely making progress. You wouldn't deny the fact that science and technology have made the world much more livable, would you," she added coyly.

Yoga for the New Millennium 85

Sanatan Swami did not agree. "Actually, the world has become increasingly unlivable: industrial waste, river pollution, nuclear sewage, atmospheric depletion, satellite debris—the planet is becoming an industrial garbage dump, uninhabitable! And you're trying to tell us that industrialization is improving our lives? The planet is literally dying due to so-called progress." The sudden vigor of the Swami's response hushed the room.

David and Ann looked at each other, paused, and then laughed nervously. Of course the quality of life had improved, hadn't it? David directed a question to Kuang Shi. "Would anyone in China not want industrialization? To be able to travel to work in one's own car or in a subway, rather than pedaling for hours on a bicycle? To have a television? Who wouldn't want a refrigerator to keep his food fresh?" Without waiting for an answer he looked at Sanatan Swami. "The benefits that have been gained by industrialization are accepted by every sane person in the world."

But Sanatan Swami was not convinced. "Industrialization may provide more leisure time, but how is that time going to be utilized? It's debatable whether there actually is more time. People are working just as hard now as they did a hundred years ago. Previously everyone was employed, whereas now there is massive unemployment. Idle and dissatisfied, people are turning to crime to replace respectable means of livelihood. The *Bhagavad-gītā* describes such persons in this way:

> Taking shelter of insatiable lust, pride and false prestige, and being thus illusioned, the demoniac are always sworn to unclean work, attracted by the impermanent. They believe that to gratify the senses is the prime necessity of human civilization. Thus until the end of life their anxiety is immeasurable. Bound by a network of hundreds of thousands of desires

and absorbed in lust and anger, they secure money by illegal means for sense gratification.

"This is a description of the godless. They don't know the goal of life, nor do they believe in life after death. Instead, they become enamored of temporary possessions like their property, family, land, and bank balance, not realizing that whatever they have is due simply to good deeds performed in past lives. Ignorant of the law of karma or, to put it simply, cause and effect, demoniac persons, although rich, well-educated, or beautiful, think that all these are merely accidental or due solely to their personal abilities. And this demoniac nature is confirmed when they immediately turn on you and become enemies, if anyone tries to interfere with their enjoyment. The result, we can all see, is that enmity and war break out among individuals and countries. It's literally a vicious cycle, and modern industrialization is both the effect of demoniac qualities and the cause of yet more. As the *Gītā* emphasizes, this is the grand illusion, and each thinks that he is God and can do anything he damn well pleases."

"Whew!" Winston gasped. "Heavy." And as if saying the thing which was on everyone's mind at the same moment, he added, "Don't you think that you're being rather uncompromising?" He thought for a moment. "I mean, no one's that bad; I mean, what you've just said applies to all of us. Are we demons?" They all nodded at Winston, giving their tacit approval to what he had said.

Sanatan Swami smiled and said, "Don't take it personally. Obviously you're not demons or you wouldn't be here. The vast majority of people, however, do fit these descriptions in one way or another. As far as they are concerned there is no God. There is only man and his potential for conquering over the laws of nature. But despite all their efforts, nature refuses to be conquered." Sanatan Swami turned to Kuang Shi. "In China, every May, there is mass flooding with great loss of life and property. Yet, by August severe drought sets in, causing equally severe suffering. Little do they realize that their sinful activities are the actual cause of these disturbances."

Winston then said, "Well, I'm glad to learn that we're not all that bad. But could you please clarify that last point. I mean about the relationship between man's sinful activities and the reactions of nature."

"It's not difficult to understand. I'll give you a practical example: If you fail to pay your electric or water bill, what happens?"

"The city turns off the supply."

"Precisely. In the same way, man is being punished for refusing to pay for nature's provisions. And how do you pay? By worshiping God. As explained in the *Bhagavad-gītā*:

> All living bodies subsist on food grains, which are produced from rains. Rains are produced by performance of sacrifice, and sacrifice is born of prescribed duties.

"In other words, we have to depend on the production of the fields, not the factories. The foods necessary for human society like food grains, vegetables, fruits, etc., and even the animals which eat these grains and vegetables, cannot be manufactured by industrial enterprise. The immeasurable quantity of water and sunshine needed to produce the world's food needs can be supplied only by nature—and nature is under the control of the Supreme Lord."

"Now, let me understand you correctly on this," Winston persisted. "Do you actually mean to say that worshiping God will solve all the world's food problems?"

"Yes."

Carlos sprang forward to the edge of his seat. "In my country nearly everyone believes in God, but that hasn't kept them from starving."

"There's a difference between vague belief and the science of devotion."

"What about overpopulation?" asked Red.

"It's a myth!" Everyone laughed.

"A myth?!" repeated David with disbelief. "Are you serious?"

"Quite serious," said Sanatan Swami gravely. "There is enough land on this planet to feed more than ten times the world's population, despite regional food shortages, and many experts have confirmed it. The real problem is mismanagement. While in Africa and Asia people are starving, elsewhere millions of tons of food are dumped into the ocean to keep market prices artificially inflated. Throughout the world there's so much land lying fallow. While cities become overpopulated, festering with problems, there aren't enough farmers to cultivate all the land. People starve, while their land is used instead to grow coffee, tea, and graze cattle for slaughter—all for the sake of earning foreign revenue.

"In the *Bhagavad-gītā*, Krishna declares Himself to be the father of all living beings. God is not a poor man, incapable of looking after His children. His opulence is unlimited. We don't find other living creatures starving. Overpopulation is a theory concocted to conceal the sin of mismanagement. And what's worse, people have been misled to believe that eating animal flesh is the only means to obtain the protein necessary for good health, though there are alternatives which are much more economical. Cultivating soy beans, for example, yields twenty times the amount of protein that an identical piece of land supplies when used for cattle raising."

"Are you vegetarians?" David inquired.

"Yes—but more than that, we eat what can be offered to Krishna: milk products, fruits, grains, beans, nuts, as well as vegetables."

"They're expert at cooking," Kuang Shi said with a broad smile.

"You've got to visit their center on a Sunday when they have their feasts," confirmed Red. "It's as good as anything you can get in the best restaurants in New York."

David followed up his previous question. "Do you follow a vegetarian diet for religious reasons?"

"No, for scientific reasons. Here's what the *Bhagavad-gītā* says about the effects of eating different types of foods:

> Foods dear to those in the mode of goodness increase the duration of life, purify one's existence and give strength, health, happiness, and satisfaction. Such foods are juicy, fatty, wholesome, and pleasing to the heart.
>
> Foods that are too bitter, too sour, salty, hot, pungent, dry and burning are dear to those in the mode of passion. Such foods cause distress, misery and disease.
>
> Food prepared more than three hours before being eaten, food that is tasteless, decomposed and putrid, and food consisting of remnants and untouchable things is dear to those in the mode of ignorance.

"There's no need of eating meat, fish, or eggs. The necessary animal protein and fat are readily available in milk products without killing innocent creatures. Don't you see, by constantly slaughtering defenseless animals, we become cruel and hard-hearted, and it's this same lack of compassion which allows us to slaughter our fellow human beings." Sanatan Swami looked at them. "If by religious you mean merciful, then yes, we are vegetarians. Mercifulness, truthfulness, austerity, and cleanliness are qualities esteemed by all religions. It is these religious qualities which differentiate man from all other creatures."

"Uh, I don't mean to interrupt you, Maharaj; but putting aside the moral issues for a moment, I can't see how eating meat, fish, or eggs is unscientific." Winston reached through his thick beard to scratch his chin. "Besides," he said, smiling affably, "I like the way they taste."

"Ananta, why don't you explain the physiological differences between a human body and that of other animals." He relaxed for a moment while his disciple spoke.

"When we look at the stomach of the human body," the student said, "it's obvious that it's not at all suited to eating meat."

"Really? It seems pretty suitable to me," said Winston, still carrying on jovially and tapping his rounded belly.

"Yes, tap your stomach, because there lies the answer. Your intestines are twelve times longer than your body, but in meat-eating animals they're only three times as long. Meat rots so quickly that it has to be eliminated from the body quickly before it becomes toxic. Creatures with short intestinal tracts have no problems digesting meat, but for man it is the source of so many diseases. The Journal of the American Medical Association reports that nearly all heart disease can be prevented by a vegetarian diet."

"Really?" Winston grew noticeably less jolly.

"Furthermore, meat-eaters have claws and sharp front teeth for tearing animal flesh." He reached over and took hold of Winston's hand. "No claws."

"At least not yet!" chuckled Red.

"There are other differences as well to prove that man is not a meat-eater. Animals that eat meat perspire through their tongues rather than their skin pores. When the food reaches their stomach, it is digested by strong hydrochloric acid, while the acid in man's stomach is twenty times less strong. Animals like the monkey, cow, and horse, which eat only vegetables, fruits, or grains, have physiological characteristics similar to man's in regard to digestion."

"What about karma?" asked Red, with a knowing look. "Tell them what the long-range effects of eating meat are. You know, in the next life." Having visited the Hare Krishna center a number of times, Red had asked the question for the sake of the others.

"Let Kuang Shi answer," said the teacher.

Kuang Shi recalled their meeting, when he had asked a similar question. With deliberate care, he repeated to the best of his remembrance, "For killing another creature you have to suffer the fate of being killed in the same way in your next birth." He looked toward the teacher to see if he had made any mistake.

"Well, that's a relief," sighed Winston. "I only eat meat. I've never killed an animal in my life," he said with a smirk.

"It's the same thing, Winston. Whether or not you kill the animal personally doesn't matter. The point is, you had something to do with the animal's death." Kuang Shi's conviction surprised everyone.

Sanatan Swami elaborated, "The *Vedas* describe animal killing as murder. Whether one feeds the animal for the purpose of fattening it, or later on performs the actual killing, cleans the carcass, delivers it, cooks it, serves it, or ultimately feeds on it, all are equally guilty and are punishable by the laws of karma."

"Changing the subject, may I know your views on abortion?" inquired Ann respectfully.

"It's not really a different subject, because abortion is also murder. The fetus in the womb is certainly alive, isn't it? It's futile to argue that it's 'less alive,' because it's still sustained by the mother. Sometimes patients are put on mechanical life support systems. Would anyone think of pulling the plug and killing the patient?"

"Some would," commented Red. "There's growing support for mercy killing. Many consider it an act of compassion to allow those with no hope of survival an early death."

"But the fetus in the womb is not at all hopeless. Left alone, it will one day be born and enjoy a full life. Abortion is a clear signal that mankind has fallen to a condition lower than any animal."

"I don't see how you can say that," Ann protested. "There are compelling factors which may lead to the decision for abortion. The mother's life may be at risk, or she may be the victim of rape. Or a family may simply not be able to afford having another child."

"If they can't afford it, they should never have conceived the child in the first place," responded Sanatan Swami sternly.

"It's not always possible to control everything," Carlos blurted out. He had been silently, almost pensively listening to the discussion. "In my country I have seen women not yet fifteen years old with three or four babies. What kind of future is that? The husband has left them or has been killed in a war. To grow up in such conditions is pure hell."

"And your answer," said Sanatan Swami boldly, "is to kill them! That's no solution. First, you should understand the cause of the problem. The cause..."

"The cause is power politics," said Carlos angrily. "Greed! To benefit a few, millions suffer."

"Carlos is not altogether wrong," Kuang Shi said sympathetically. "Recently I read a report from China that prostitution, which plagued China before Liberation, is making a strong comeback, especially in some urban areas. The report noted that in a particular place, Shenzhen, a special economic zone for foreign investors, the many factories have attracted a large number of women workers. Due to the vastly disproportionate number of women, prostitution, homosexuality, and divorce are becoming increasing problems. Naturally there will be abortions in such situations."

"It's not at all natural," stated the spiritual master. "In a natural agrarian economy such problems would never have arisen. These are the effects of rapid industrialization, problems that are commonplace in developed nations. People think there is no alternative. As long as the leaders fail to realize that the real goal of human life is self-realization and not sense-gratification, these problems will only increase. In Vedic times the leaders were not only administrators, they were sages as well. They could never have imagined allowing abortion. Even animals at least wait until their offspring are born before they kill them. But now we have become better than the animals, because we don't have to wait for our offspring to be born before we kill them. In some countries women are given bonuses and paid vacations for having an abortion."

"The latest business is fetus harvesting." Everyone listened attentively as Red continued. "Ann and Charlie would probably know about this. It's part of genetic engineering, which aims to make things grow faster and mature more quickly by changing the genetic code. Of course as with any experiment, there have been problems. Programming changes into the biological codes without first fully understanding how the organisms relate in the overall delicate balance of nature creates insuperable problems. For example they have placed human genes into the permanent genetic code of pigs to make them grow larger. Unfortunately, the pigs developed arthritis, cross-eyedness, and some were born without anuses and other essential parts. Can you imagine placing a growth hormone gene into a human egg or sperm and making humans that grow twice as big or twice as fast for the rest of history?" Red had succeeded in doing what he was best at—completely capturing everyone's attention.

Kuang Shi was becoming a bit nervous, knowing Red's tendency to dominate a situation. "What about 'fetal harvesting,' " he said, hoping to remind Red of his original topic.

"I'm getting to that. Now with the ability to cross boundaries between species by placing genes from one animal to another, the business community is becoming alert to a huge commercial potential. As a result the United States Patent Office said that all animals on the planet can now be patented, except of course humans."

"They'll be next," said Winston with a laugh.

"Playing God," Sanatan Swami stated. "This is the final delusion of material science. After reducing life to mere chemicals, they now want to reduce it even further to information codes that can be simulated on the computer and redefined to produce a new creation all their own. They will simply create chaos." Everyone was silent. "And fetus harvesting?"

"Yes," Red continued, "they're using the organs and tissues of aborted fetuses for research as well as the tissues for implanting into needy patients. One television commentator suggested that this could lead to women becoming factories for producing human fetuses for medical experimentation."

"Horrible!" said Winston, aghast. There was a long silence.

Sanatan Swami quickly surveyed the group. Youthful optimism had been appalled by the grotesqueries of human vision run amok. He was not shocked by what he had heard, though he could see that they were. Collective humanity was going mad. Red Simon was struck by the notion of Pandora's box and the parable of evil unleashed upon the world, whereas Winston remembered stories he had heard about Nazi concentration camp experiments and wondered if the Third Reich had survived after all.

The phrase "nuclear mutants" tumbled over and over again in Ann's mind. As Carlos sat biting his nails. Kuang Shi looked over at Sanatan Swami, who was deep in thought: "... bound by hundreds of thousands of illicit desires, they were sworn to sinful activity." The words of the *Bhagavad-gītā* came to his mind:

> Those who are demoniac do not know what is to be done and what is not to be done. Neither cleanliness nor proper behavior nor truth is found in them. They say that this world is unreal, with no foundation, no God in control. They say it is produced of sex desire and has no cause other than lust. Following such conclusions, the demoniac, who are lost to themselves and who have no intelligence, engage in unbeneficial, horrible works meant to destroy the world.

This brief conversation had further affirmed his realization that there was a single underlying cause to all the world's problems: a total lack of God consciousness. The *Bhagavad-gītā* had the solution: the only question was how to convince them.

"My friends," he began, "you look surprised. Without education how do you expect people to behave properly? What you're witnessing is nothing more than animalism. An animal has no goal other than sense gratification. Demoniac, animal-like men cannot comprehend the fact that human life means but one thing, to free oneself from the pain of birth, old age, disease, and death. Unfortunately, ignorant men are busy trying to fulfill their temporary plans, which only result in their own destruction and cast them back down into the vicious cycle of birth and death."

"Fine," David said, "then suggest some practical program to help others?"

"First one must help oneself." Sanatan Swami began, but before he could finish, Carlos leaned forward and cut him off. "That's just another kind of selfishness, thinking only of oneself while others suffer is not my idea of compassion."

"Then why did you come to America?" retorted the Swami, returning the challenge. "Because by improving yourself you hope to be able to help your countrymen in the future. Am I right?" Carlos' slight, tan body remained tense at the edge of his seat. He remained silent, tight-lipped. Sanatan Swami continued. "People don't see that they're suffering. So dulled are they by their difficulties, they concoct all kinds of makeshift solutions. But this is not the standard of happiness, which means but one thing, the cessation of all suffering."

"That's Utopian," Ann said. Although she had appreciated the many points made by the learned master, she was skeptical of any positive alternatives.

"For one who has remained in prison his entire life, to be a free citizen seems Utopian. We have been thrown into the prison of material existence for so many lifetimes that we can't remember what it's like to be free. But when one achieves Krishna consciousness he experiences his original blissful state."

"Is there some practical method for achieving it?"

"I'm glad you asked. Are any of you familiar with chanting Hare Krishna? Ananta, don't we have a *bhakti-yoga* club established here?"

"There is one," said Winston. "I've attended a number of meetings. We're all familiar with Hare Krishna. Everyone in New York is."

"But have any of you actually tried chanting?" Noting their silence, Sanatan Swami indicated that Ananta should give each a *mantra* card. After explaining its meaning he suggested they try chanting together. Playing a small set of hand cymbals, he led the chanting: Hare Krishna, Hare Krishna, Krishna Krishna, Hare Hare/Hare

Rama, Hare Rama, Rama Rama, Hare Hare.

Kuang Shi found the second time chanting much easier than the first. He already knew the *mantra*, so he could concentrate more on the sound. The cymbals and melody were new. He guessed that these made the chanting more appealing, though he found that they also helped him concentrate.

Ann became absorbed in the chanting. It was not new for her, though she had not mentioned anything when asked. One of her close friends who lived in California had been practicing Krishna consciousness for a number of years, and they had talked about it in their letters. But this was the first time she had chanted with others. It felt good, and the more she chanted, the more she liked it.

Winston's eyes were closed, his head swaying to the melodic chanting. He had already experimented with various types of meditation. His deep baritone voice was easily distinguishable.

Red Simon tapped his foot in time to the beat, which went one, two, three, with a strong accent on the third beat. He liked music of any type, and though he could appreciate that the chanting was far more than just another pop song, for the moment he was singing along mostly because he liked the way it sounded. David was a bit hesitant. He would chant, only slightly moving his lips, then look up self-consciously to see what the others were doing.

Carlos didn't even try. For him it was religious, and the world had had enough of that. It wasn't going to put food in the mouth of his countrymen nor provide homes for the poor. Besides, his family had its own religion.

After nearly ten minutes, Sanatan Swami gave the cymbals a final strike, and the chanting ended, engulfing the room in silence. Winston was the first to speak.

"Is Krishna consciousness only a mental adjustment?" Winston wanted to know.

"No, it's a change of consciousness, in fact, a complete change of identity. At present we have misidentified ourselves with the body and thus we suffer or enjoy whatever fate befalls our body. But one who is Krishna conscious correctly identifies himself as the soul and thus enjoys continuous happiness on the spiritual platform." Sanatan Swami snapped his fingers. "I'll give you a striking example which, though it may seem odd, will indicate just how different spiritual and material consciousness really are. As a drunk does not notice that he's wearing a coat or shirt, one who is self-realized and is established in his eternal identity doesn't notice whether his external body is sitting or standing. In fact if by God's will the body dies, and if by God's will he gains a new body, the self-realized soul isn't bewildered, just as a drunken man is oblivious to the situation of his outward dress."

"A type of transcendental absentmindedness, it sounds like," joked Winston.

Ann looked at her watch. She had a report to complete and it was getting late. "Well, this has been a pleasantly refreshing evening. I'm afraid I'll have to be excusing myself."

Sanatan Swami could sense that it was the proper time to conclude the meeting. The others were also getting restless. "Before anyone leaves I'd like to invite all of you to visit our cultural center this coming Sunday. As Red confirmed, our feasts are hard to beat."

"What time Sunday?" asked Winston.

"At 4:00 p.m. Kuang Shi, why don't you organize the visit for everyone."

"Where exactly is it?" asked Kuang Shi. Ananta quickly indicated the address on the *mantra* card.

"It's only a few minutes away by subway," said Red. "Come on, Carlos, what are you doing Sunday?"

"Well, I'll have to see."

By now everyone was standing. Kuang Shi looked toward Ann. "Will you be free on Sunday?"

"I hope so. I'd very much like to come."

"We'll be there." said David, shaking Sanatan Swami's hand.

"I very much enjoyed the discussion."

"So did we all, Maharaj. Didn't we, Carlos?" said Winston to the slight Nicaraguan as he cuffed him on the shoulder. They walked down the hallway together exchanging farewells.

After escorting Sanatan Swami and Ananta to the subway entrance, Kuang Shi returned to his dormitory. He was feeling satisfied with the way everything had turned out. So many interesting topics, and so lively. All his friends had been respectful toward Sanatan Swami, except perhaps for Carlos. Sanatan Swami had complimented Kuang Shi for having such nice friends.

Upon reaching his room, Kuang Shi found a calling card which was tacked to his door. It bore the name of Dr. Zhang Chong Shu , and below the name, the title "President, Chinese People's Association for Scientific Exchange." On the bottom of the card was a Beijing address. Kuang Shi turned the card over but found the same information repeated in Chinese, with the addition of a brief note, also in Chinese, "Will phone tomorrow."

Kuang Shi could not recall having heard of the organization, nor was he acquainted with any Dr. Zhang. He wondered what the purpose of the visit might be. He'd find out tomorrow. For tonight, he'd recline in an easy chair and read the *Bhagavad-gītā*.

9

KUANG SHI'S FRIENDS differed in their perception of the meeting with Sanatan Swami. Born in the northern state of Wisconsin, Winston grew up a farmer's son. He jumped at the opportunity to go to one of America's top schools, but coming to New York had been quite a shock for the backwoods Winston. He would have felt safer lost in the forest in the middle of the night than he did walking the streets of predatory New York in broad daylight. A hungry pack of wolves was less fearsome than meeting a crazy gang of teenagers high on drugs. For one accustomed to the ambling pace of the Midwest, the frenzy with which most New Yorkers conducted their affairs would make even the sanest man neurotic. And then there was that fierce competition at school. He found himself changing his major three times—from physics to psychology to history—before finally settling on philosophy. At least he could find some direction by studying others' explanations of a world which he now perceived had somehow gone wrong. Like many of his friends, he was pessimistic about its future, and he expressed that concern by making special endeavors for personal improvement. He felt a strong inclination toward Chinese philosophy and culture, having made it his area of concentration. He developed a fascination for things Chinese: he learned the language, frequented Chinese restaurants, practiced *tai chi*, and finally upon graduation spent three months touring China.

It was natural that Winston and Kuang Shi had become close friends. Kuang Shi felt that Winston could understand him more than any other American he had met. As Kuang Shi straddled two worlds, so he also felt did Winston. The two had thus developed a close relationship. When Kuang Shi became excited upon meeting Sanatan

Swami, Winston immediately became interested. He had great respect for Kuang Shi's intelligence, but though he thought he knew him well, he was taken completely by surprise when Kuang Shi expressed his appreciation for *yoga* philosophy. Kuang Shi had always been pragmatic as much as Winston was philosophical. He had always been materialistic, while Winston would try to see the spiritual side of things. But now, for the first time, it was Kuang Shi who took the lead, steering their conversations toward a topic he would never before have been interested in. Winston became eager to meet the person who had so influenced his friend.

He had not been disappointed. He saw in the Swami a highly developed spiritual personality, the likes of which he had read about only in books. He had hoped to one day meet a genuine spiritual teacher, one he could totally trust in and take guidance from. After the initial meeting with Sanatan Swami, he had a hunch that he had finally met such a person.

Ann Denton had always preferred being alone. It gave her more time to concentrate on matters which she found most interesting. What was the use of endless parties, school dances, and movies? She found these boring in comparison with her intellectual pursuits. Aside from her family, her only real friend was David Hunt.

They had grown up in a small town in Connecticut, where everyone knew practically everyone else. David Hunt's family was the richest in town. His uncle had been a state senator, and the family could trace its prominent ancestry back many generations. Dr. Denton, Ann's father, was the family's physician.

David and Ann had gone to the same schools since they were children, but it was only in high school that they had gotten to know each other. Though they were different in many ways, the very differences seemed to attract each to the other. Their families were pleased with the thought that one day the two might get married, for David and Ann were a handsome couple. Though it was fashionable for students to date others, neither wanted to. Ann was satisfied with the arrangement, which gave her time to concentrate on her research work. As far as David was concerned, he had simply made up his mind that he would marry her.

When the time came for them to choose which college they would attend, both decided in favor of Columbia. It was one of the most prestigious in the country, and while being near to home, it was distant enough to allow them a bit of independence.

Kuang Shi had first met Ann while doing some research work in the medical school lab. Being in related fields, they had occasion to discuss their work. She was impressed by his intelligence and self-discipline and admired how for days he could focus his entire attention on a particular subject and not allow anything to distract him. Kuang Shi equally respected Ann. Unlike from so many other American women, he did not perceive any sexual intentions from her. Thus they developed a close relationship as co-researchers and even worked on some joint projects together.

When Kuang Shi invited her to meet Sanatan Swami, Ann preferred not to mention her acquaintance with the Krishna movement. In fact, it was something she had not even discussed with David. It had begun about three years ago when one of her college friends had moved to San Francisco to do graduate work at the University of California at Berkeley. She had begun receiving literature in the mail from her friend and simply kept it aside because she had so much of her own work to do. But one day a small book arrived that caught her attention. It was the same one that Kuang Shi had first received. Easy Journey to

Other Planets. She was fascinated by the title, and as she began to read it she became amazed in much the same way Kuang Shi had. As a scientist she appreciated the logical arguments of the book, realizing that they were as scientific as the theories of her school texts. The philosophy of Krishna consciousness intrigued her, and with new interest she began to read the other books her friend had sent her. Because the conclusions differed in many ways from those held by her teachers, she decided to remain silent for the time being. By the time of the meeting with Sanatan Swami, she had developed a genuine appreciation for the Vedic teachings, though there were certain doubts that still lingered in her mind. She saw the meeting as an opportunity to clear up some of these. According to her understanding, Sanatan Swami embodied all the qualities of a spiritually advanced soul as she had read about them in the *Vedas*.

The night after the meeting she dreamt she met Sanatan Swami. They chanted Hare Krishna together for what seemed forever, and when she awoke she felt a happiness she had never experienced before. Clinging to her joy she immediately began to chant and kept it up, silently when absolutely necessary, that whole day. She was therefore eagerly waiting for Sunday when she would again be able to meet the Krishna Swami.

Of all those who had attended the program, Red Simon was the only native of New York City. Born to a poor immigrant family, the eighth of ten children, Rutherford (or Red, as his friends preferred) always excelled in school. He graduated high school with top honors and was offered a full scholarship to Columbia. Anyone who had known his family background might have been surprised, but those who knew him well sensed that he was destined for great intellectual achievements.

There was no doubt in his mind as to what his major would be. What astonished everyone was his enrolling in the school of business. After graduation, he immediately went to work for a stock brokerage firm. The many connections he had made at school and at work allowed him to gain the confidence of influential persons. With their financial help he made a number of successful investments, and now, five years later, finishing his graduate studies, his net worth was well over a million dollars.

He knew when to take risks and when to be conservative. It was in his blood. There was an element of adventure in everything he did, even when he moved outside the field of business. To him, life was a challenge: sometimes he won, sometimes he lost. It was a question of averages and there was no sense becoming upset at the outcome.

This curiously ambivalent nature inclined Red toward Eastern philosophy with its concept of *yang* and *yin* that emphasized unity-in-diversity. He found the law of *karma* quite congenial, needing little encouragement to be convinced that his abilities were God-given, something he had inherited from a past life. He was too alert an observer of human destiny not to discern that fortune, whether good or bad, was never blind. Everything had its cause, and whatever could not be traced in this lifetime undoubtedly had its origin in the past one.

Red had no difficulty understanding the Krishna conscious philosophy when he first read one of their books. He had visited their center on occasion and enjoyed the chanting accompanied by music and dancing. But whereas they saw the ultimate goal to leave this world and return to a spiritual world of Krishna, he saw the repetition of birth and death as an endless cycle, and like any true gambler, you had to learn to take your losses with as much grace as the gains. In his opinion, the Krishnas were a bit too idealistic.

Carlos Hernandez was the son of a wealthy plantation owner and grew up in the tense atmosphere of bitter class struggle. Like so many Latin-American countries, Nicaragua had been a U.S. supported dictatorship in which a few select families controlled nearly all the land, resources, and wealth of the country. It was a country in which class distinctions meant everything, one's personal abilities very little. Carlos' birth assured him a life of ease and servants to do practically every conceivable chore, so that life for the family, other than the father's indirect overseeing of their vast properties, consisted of a gay social life shared with similarly wealthy families. He had his own horses and went to the best of schools; in short, he was able to have everything that money could buy.

The fact that his family's fortunes were absolutely dependent on the sufferings of others was unbearable to him. For young Carlos it made no sense, and as he grew up he found the inequities still more unacceptable. If his life had been a series of contradictions, there was no dilemma greater than that which he felt at present. Here he was, taking shelter in America—taking advantage of its educational, economic, cultural, and political institutions—while the very same America was now waging war on his countrymen. For Carlos, his life had become an unbearable hypocrisy. But what could he do? He found himself in the same dilemma he had throughout his life, incapable of doing anything about a situation vastly beyond his control.

At least he could prepare for the future. He majored in political science, with the hope that one day statesmanship and his understanding of world history and the trends which shaped key events would be of service to his countrymen. While in America, he decided to help Latin Americans gain their rights and became politically active in a number of New York minority groups. He worked with young drug addicts. He felt that these were practical ways in which he could help alleviate suffering in the world.

He befriended Kuang Shi, seeing him as a representative of the most important communist nation in the world. China, to him, was a symbol of what a nation could accomplish once it freed itself of foreign and local suppression. Though Kuang Shi had little interest in Carlos' polemics, out of politeness he gave him a patient hearing and appreciated his great sincerity. Carlos would ask endless questions about China, but when Kuang Shi described the present reforms Carlos seemed surprised, even disappointed.

Due to his friendship with Kuang Shi and Winston he had agreed to come to the *yoga* meeting. Otherwise he saw little benefit to such meditational methods, which he viewed as more or less selfishly motivated. He had tried to read the book which Kuang Shi had given him, but found it dull and uninteresting.

Dr. Zhang, the President of the Chinese People's Association for Scientific Exchange, had made an appointment to see Kuang Shi on Thursday morning. Dr. Zhang was elderly, somewhere in his seventies, but he was not frail, as Li Kuang Shi quickly found out from his firm handshake. He was immaculately dressed, slim, shorter than Li Kuang Shi, and nearly bald. They sat down in the easy chairs exchanging pleasantries in Chinese. Kuang Shi poured his visitor a cup of tea.

"May I know your field of study, Dr. Zhang?" inquired Kuang Shi politely.

"I am no longer actively engaged in research. My work with the association absorbs me full-time, but my background is in biochemistry, as is yours." Dr. Zhang smiled pleasantly. Kuang Shi wondered what else his visitor knew about him.

"You must have opportunity to visit many countries?"

"Oh yes, many. In fact, I served in Geneva for several years as a member of the World Health Organization." Dr. Zhang looked at Li Kuang Shi thoughtfully, and then quickly came to the point. "No doubt you are wondering why I have come. You have been in America for five years, so you must be accustomed to their ways. While we Chinese are more ceremonious and formal, they prefer frankness. The Chinese government has been following your progress with great satisfaction. Have you been awarded your doctorate yet?"

"My thesis was approved," said Li Kuang Shi, listening intently.

"We are very pleased you have chosen to specialize in the study of human immune deficiency viruses. The problem of AIDS is a worldwide concern, and already a number of cases have been diagnosed in China involving foreigners. We expect that the problem will only increase as tourism continues to grow. Our nation is no longer insulated from the world as it was for so many years. With increasing contact on all levels, there is no way we can avoid this problem."

"What steps is the Chinese government taking in regard to research?"

"Not as much as we would like to. As you are well aware, it is a new problem. In fact, I was in France when the first AIDS diagnosis was made public there. Even the United States began research only 2 years ago, in 1986 and is still behind some of the European countries."

"The problem here is that the issue has become so publicized, it becomes difficult for researchers to find privacy to do their work. They're constantly being spotlighted and interviewed. Everyone is asking, 'Is there a cure?' As if the issue were such an easy one." He looked directly at Dr. Zhang. "It remains an open question whether a vaccine is at all possible."

"If it is, it will be discovered by someone like yourself."

Kuang Shi laughed. "I'm just a student, a mere novice in

the field. The top men in this country, heads of institutions like the National Institute of Allergy and Infectious Diseases and the Center for Disease Control are putting their full energy into it."

"But you have the background. You've done intensive studies in genetics and molecular biology."

Kuang Shi could not help but be surprised.

"You know quite a bit about me, don't you. Dr. Zhang?"

"We are especially concerned with the most promising of our students, especially those who have gone overseas. There are not many Ph.D. holders in China, so your achievement is rare. Intellectuals are being shown much more respect now. Especially in the field of science, our government is trying to give special emphasis."

"Things were improving even before I left," said Kuang Shi.

"And they will continue to improve," Dr. Zhang confidently replied.

"But it is still true that those who work on missiles earn less than egg peddlers, while a surgeon who works with a scalpel earns less than a barber who works with a razor. I'm afraid that this saying is not yet outdated. How can our government expect intellectuals to be encouraged when they are plagued by housing shortages, poor health, and low salaries? How can they have the peace of mind necessary for their research?"

"We are trying our best to remedy it, but such changes cannot take place overnight. In the meantime, intellectuals should dedicate themselves to the principles of reform by supporting the government in every way. Unfortunately, many students have become enamored with the idea of going to America and other Western nations." Dr. Zhang faced Kuang Shi squarely. "Some think of not returning at all."

Kuang Shi felt the official's eyes stare directly into his

conscience. Dr. Zhang's meaning was clear.

"Money is not everything," Kuang Shi admitted.

"But it does mean a great deal, doesn't it?" It was a leading question.

"A sincere scientist is concerned for the welfare of others, not for his personal aggrandizement. We are living in a small world, Dr. Zhang. Scientific research and knowledge are not like military secrets. Countries like America have so much to give to poor countries like ours. The kind of research that can be done here would be very difficult there. Especially in fields like mine, which require sophisticated equipment and tremendous interdepartmental coordination. It would be very difficult to duplicate my research work in China."

"So you admit you intend to stay here."

Kuang Shi was silent for a moment. "I have not admitted to anything personally." he said evasively. "I have simply stated factually what would be true for anyone in my field."

"How much money have you been offered to stay here?" The question was a blunt one. "Are you only interested in money like so many others?" he challenged.

Kuang Shi remained silent. Dr. Zhang was elderly and he therefore respected him.

"Those of us who are especially fortunate must not forget our people." Dr. Zhang's words immediately reminded Kuang Shi of Sanatan Swami's telling him, "One who receives this knowledge bears a great responsibility. I'm not simply speaking for your sake. I am thinking of your Chinese brothers and sisters. Do you understand?"

"I came to make you an offer." Though he did not look up. Kuang Shi listened carefully. "We want to establish an AIDS research department. It will be connected to the People's Liberation Army General Hospital and will receive special funding. You will be given the position of chief of research."

Kuang Shi was now looking directly at Dr. Zhang. With some effort he managed to say, "I am honored."

"A special fund has been set aside to purchase the most up-to-date equipment. A special building has already been allocated. There will be others also of similar background as yours, as well as large support staff. Of course we cannot offer you the kind of money you could make here, but as you said, money isn't everything." He smiled, and then added, "Is it, Dr. Li?" After a moment's pause, "I know you will want some time to consider all this. Perhaps you were making other plans which would have to change now."

"When were you thinking to start this new department, Dr. Zhang?"

"Toward the end of the summer, Dr. Li. In Beijing I know the weather is very fine at that time. Do you sometimes remember your home?"

"One never forgets one's home, Dr. Zhang."

"I'll allow you to return to your work. I'm glad that we had this meeting. I am sorry you couldn't have dinner with me. I know a lovely restaurant I would have taken you to. Perhaps next time. But then, next time may be in Beijing." He smiled suggestively, gave Kuang Shi a firm handshake, and left quickly.

10

KUANG SHI LOOKED AT his watch. It was nearly 4:00 P.M. His habit was always to be on time. No sooner had they turned the corner of Schermerhorn Street and Nevins Street when they spotted their destination.

"There's the building!" said Red, pointing to an impressive stone and brick building. As they approached the building they noticed a number of cars stopping in front of it. When they entered they were surprised to find themselves in a large, well-decorated lobby with hundreds of persons milling about. It distinctly reminded one of a busy hotel lobby. Crystal chandeliers hung elegantly overhead. On the walls hung paintings of philosophical themes as well as portraits of great spiritual personalities.

Kuang Shi wondered how they would find Ananta. Looking about he noticed an information desk. He was about to approach a young lady dressed in an Indian sari when he heard Ananta's voice calling his name from a distance.

"I'm sorry," Ananta said, running up excitedly. "I was setting up the sound system for Sanatan Swami's lecture. Have you been waiting long?"

"No, we just arrived," replied Kuang Shi, feeling relieved to meet their host. "I never expected that there would be so many people."

"There'll be at least two or three thousand guests before the evening is over. It's like this every Sunday."

"Do the same people come every weekend?" Kuang Shi asked, impressed.

"At least a third are like you, persons coming for the first time. They've read our books, maybe attended one of our seminars, or have been invited by a member."

"Perhaps some of them visited your Festival of India just as I did," Kuang Shi observed.

"Follow me," said Ananta, weaving his way to the rear corner of the lobby. "You'll have to take your shoes off here." He directed them to the shoe room. This is similar to Buddhist temple tradition, Kuang Shi thought. Walking in his stocking feet, he noticed for the first time the marble floors, polished to a mirror-like finish.

"Get ready for a surprise!" Red exclaimed as they passed through a narrow hallway. They were completely unprepared for the sight as Ananta led them into a vast, dazzlingly ornate hall.

"Incredible!" said Winston. The richness of the decorations left everyone speechless. The entire hall was radiant with an iridescent light, as the afternoon sunshine flowing through tinted glass was refracted into myriad colors and mirrored in the shiny floor, which was made of rich Italian marbles cut and arranged in patterns of pink and yellow lotus flowers against a blue background. The walls were covered by magnificent, sculptured murals, perhaps twenty feet in height and thirty feet in length, depicting scenes from the *Bhagavad-gītā*. Each was separated by finely carved marble pillars that reached two-thirds of the way toward the ceiling to the stained glass windows.

An assembly of more than a thousand sat quietly on individual cushions. Many of them were softly repeating the *mantra*: Hare Krishna, Hare Krishna, Krishna Krishna, Hare Hare / Hare Rama, Hare Rama, Rama Rama, Hare Hare. Those who were not seated gathered at the front of the hall at the foot of a raised, stage-like inner room. It was even more brilliantly lit and ornate than the main hall and contained a shrine which seemed to be made of gold and silver. Within the shrine stood two statues, one black, the other white, which appeared to be the focal point of everyone's devotion. Some stood praying with folded palms, while others bowed low, touching their foreheads to the floor.

At the opposite end of the hall stood a smaller structure, enthroning a life-size statue of someone who resembled the Buddha.

"Who's that?" inquired Mary. "How can he sit so still?"

Red had been to the temple a number of times and explained, "It's only a statue. It's their founder."

Ananta confirmed, "His Divine Grace A.C. Bhaktivedanta Swami Prabhupāda, the founder of our worldwide society."

Kuang Shi recognized the name as the translator and commentator of the *Bhagavad-gītā As It Is*. He watched as worshipers bowed before the image of the revered master. The entire scene reminded Kuang Shi of a temple in Beijing he had once visited. Following the death of his grandfather, his father had taken him to make offerings on behalf of the departed soul. That temple was certainly much grander than the one in his village, where his father would take him on certain special occasions. He remembered statues of the Goddess of Mercy, the God of Wealth, the Dragon God, and the Earth God. He could not remember very much because the temple had been closed suddenly by the Red Guards, who used it as a barracks. No one knew what became of the gods.

That was the last time Kuang Shi had visited a temple, except of course when on holiday he and his college friends had once spent an afternoon at the Fayuansi temple. At the time, they looked with curiosity upon the devoted worshipers and were wondering how in this age of science people could still hold tightly to such superstitious beliefs. Even his father no longer went to any temple. In the light of modern education, the number who did was rapidly diminishing.

Kuang Shi looked at the ornately decorated architecture of the hall. It was without doubt the most beautifully adorned of any he had ever seen. But in a country where even the banks resembled palaces, such opulence was not extraordinary. Though America was the most technologically advanced nation in the world, nearly everyone believed in God and religion. When he had first come to America he was amazed at how many churches and temples existed, especially compared with China, where most had been destroyed or converted to other uses. He had always considered religion and science to be irreconcilable, but it was clear that Americans didn't.

Suddenly everyone began bowing down. They all turned to Ananta for an explanation, but he too was bowing down. Ann motioned to the far end of the hall, where they saw the strong and graceful form of Sanatan Swami enter. He wore a garland of fresh flowers. He went up to the shrine where the founder's image was seated and prostrated himself fully upon the floor before it. Rising, he walked the entire distance to the other end of the hall and did the same before the larger shrine of the black and white statues.

Sanatan Swami spotted Kuang Shi and his friends and immediately walked over to them. "I'm glad that you could come." The warmth in his greeting made them feel very happy that they had come. "But where's your friend Carlos?"

Kuang Shi said, "One of his friends had an accident and he wanted to visit the family to try to console them."

"Let me show you around the temple room. Let's walk around the side so as not to disturb the people who are meditating."

"It's just like church," Mary said. Seeing many chant on small wooden beads reminded her of Catholic rosary beads.

"Yes. There are many similarities in all religions. Buddhists also chant on the same number of beads as we do, one hundred eight."

They had reached the shrine in which the statue of the founder was seated.

"He looks so real. I thought he was alive!" said Mary unabashedly. Red realized he had not yet introduced his friend and did so. Sanatan Swami greeted her warmly and continued, 'This is the worshipable form of our founder and spiritual master of Krishna consciousness worldwide. He is my spiritual master as well."

"You mean you also have a spiritual master?" Mary

asked. Sanatan Swami seemed to appreciate the question.

"Yes, everyone must have a spiritual master, otherwise how can they learn this science of devotion?"

"Are you the spiritual master for all these people here?" said Mary wide-eyed.

Sanatan Swami smiled. "No. The relationship between the guru and disciple is personal and can't be institutionalized. Each person must find his or her own spiritual master."

"But how do you know when you've met your guru," Winston asked. "There are specific qualities by which one can identify a genuine spiritual master. The most important qualification is that he be a pure devotee of the Supreme Lord, and these qualities are described in books like the *Bhagavad-gītā*. It's no mystery. A qualified spiritual master is like a good boat captain. To cross the ocean one needs a very strong boat. The human body is such a worthy ocean-going vessel, as compared with other types of bodies, like those of the animals and lower creatures, which are like smaller boats, incapable of making an ocean-crossing. Therefore, one can cross over the ocean of ignorance and all its suffering only when one attains the human form of life. We are not experienced to navigate across the ocean on our own, but require a proper person, a captain for the ship, who knows how to take advantage of the favorable breezes, which are compared to the Vedic literatures such as the *Bhagavad-gītā*. So here is a real captain," said Sanatan Swami, indicating his spiritual master seated within the shrine.

"You are our captain, Maharaj," Winston said, his palms folded reverentially.

"When did you first meet Śrīla Prabhupāda?" Ann asked. Sanatan Swami studied her very carefully, wondering how she had known the proper title for his spiritual master.

"You know what the title 'Śrīla Prabhupāda' means?" he asked her.

"One at whose feet all masters sit," she said, as if repeating a lesson.

Sanatan Swami was visibly pleased with this young lady who had properly understood the exalted position of his divine master. Within his mind he prayed that she might become Krishna conscious. "I first met Prabhupāda shortly after he arrived from India," Sanatan Swami replied. "There were not many devotees in those days. Those were very humble beginnings. He came with only five dollars and a trunkful of his books, but from those simple beginnings this huge organization has developed, all due to his purity and prayers that the world become Krishna conscious. As a fire is kindled from wood by another fire, so the divine consciousness of men all over the world was kindled by the fire of His Divine Grace. That is known as *parampāra*, disciplic succession. As I am instructing you, so he instructed me."

Mary interjected again, "Who instructed him?"

"The knowledge we are teaching has come down over thousands of years through an unbroken line of spiritual teachers."

David had been listening, somewhat skeptically. He was stunned to hear Ann so familiar with the Krishna philosophy. After all, she had never mentioned anything of it to him. Looking at the statue in the shrine, he asked, "So what is the source of this knowledge? Where did it come from?"

"Krishna," Sanatan Swami said simply.

David wasn't satisfied. He challenged the Swami, "But who is Krishna? A God? A man? Just some myth?"

Sanatan Swami knew the consciousness of the young people standing before him. Each was on a different level of spiritual realization and required special handling. He had to choose his words carefully so they would all be satisfied. "It's not difficult to understand who Krishna is, providing one inquires properly. The *Bhagavad-gītā* describes the proper attitude for the sincere seeker:

> Just try to learn the truth by approaching a spiritual master. Inquire from him submissively and render service unto him. The self-realized souls can impart knowledge unto you because they have seen the truth.

"Have you seen the truth?" David's question was charged with emotion. Ann could not understand why David, who was normally so mild in his behavior, was being so challenging. Kuang Shi was also surprised, and Sanatan Swami too felt the tension. Rather than answer directly he decided to give an example.

"The truth can't be understood by one's own endeavor, but is revealed of its own accord. Just because you want to see the sun rise at night won't make it appear. It will rise on its own at the proper time in the morning, not on your command. We're all in the darkness of ignorance, and until we are enlightened, we cannot expect to see the truth. We have to work to become enlightened and wait for that time when the truth, of its own accord, manifests itself before us."

Kuang Shi was confused. Why didn't the master answer David directly? What did he mean by the "truth"? Everybody had his own conception of what was true and what was false. Was he speaking of some kind of absolute truth? Respectfully, he submitted his question to the learned teacher. "What do you mean by 'truth' and exactly how does one understand it?"

Sanatan Swami felt Kuang Shi's sincerity. He sensed that Kuang Shi would listen patiently, as would Ann and

Winston. David only became impatient, while Mary drifted off to the side to look at one of the large wall panels. He suggested that they sit down, because his explanation might take some time.

"According to the *Bhagavad-gītā* truth, or reality, is whatever is permanent. Whereas, whatever is temporary is considered illusory. For example, the foam on the ocean water or the clouds in the sky are temporary. The clouds produce rain, which makes the vegetation grow. But the clouds, rain, and vegetation are all temporary and will disappear in due course of time. However, the sky is permanent. The Absolute Truth is compared to the eternal sky, while the cloud-like illusions come and go. Only fools are attracted by the ephemeral, cloud-like illusions of this world, while truly intelligent men are interested in the eternal truth."

Winston grasped at the concept. "So the truth is beyond the world we live in?"

"No. The Absolute Truth is everywhere." Winston gave a puzzled look. Sanatan Swami directed his words to Kuang Shi. "The Absolute Truth is like all-pervading space. Science acknowledges that our universe is only one of many, and that all of them are situated within outer space. This impersonal aspect of the Absolute Truth is like endless space."

Winston was even more confused. "Impersonal aspect?"

"There's a personal aspect as well as an impersonal aspect of the Absolute Truth."

"What's the difference?" Winston rocked backward and forward in his seat, trying to understand.

"When astronauts go into space, the initial euphoria of floating free soon wears off, and they again desire to land. Why?"

"Why what?" Winston queried.

"They probably get bored," offered David casually.

"Exactly!" Everyone was surprised that Sanatan Swami agreed with David's offhanded remark. "They get bored with so little to do. Outside the spacecraft, there is an awesome sense of endless space, compounded by a sense of timelessness."

"Sounds horrible!" joked David. "I think I'd prefer the personal aspect of the truth myself."

Sanatan Swami and Ananta both smiled. "You'll be glad to know that the *Bhagavad-gītā* agrees with you. It's very difficult to conceive of the impersonal, or the unmanifest, that which is beyond the perception of our senses. We are persons, so it is natural for us to relate to a personal concept when we think of the Absolute Truth."

Winston spoke, "In other words, that's why people imagine God to be a person. They assign God the same qualities they themselves have." That sounded logical to Kuang Shi. He waited to see if Sanatan Swami agreed.

He did not. God was not a figment of the imagination, a creation of man. Rather, God created man in His image. "The Absolute Truth is the origin of all qualities: all beauty, wealth, knowledge, strength, fame, and renunciation are present in Him."

"But everyone has these qualities," Winston objected.

"Not unlimitedly."

David was becoming somewhat impatient. "But what is this Absolute Truth, anyway? Is it something you can see or touch? It must be, if as you say it has all those qualities."

Sanatan Swami knew that it was still unclear to them. He decided to speak more plainly. "The Absolute Truth is a person."

"A person?!" Winston was incredulous—as indeed they all were.

"An Absolute Person," Sanatan Swami said, in answer to their astonishment.

"But Maharaj, if the Absolute Truth is beginningless and all-pervading, wouldn't you be limiting it by saying that it's a person?"

Sanatan Swami sought to dispel their doubts. "I'm not speaking of an ordinary person like you or me. The Supreme Personality is fully spiritual: He sees everywhere and hears everything. Thus, He knows everything, past, present, and future."

Winston's eyes grew wide. "Okay, okay, how do I get to meet Him?"

David picked up on the humor. "Where does He live? And even if you did meet Him, would you recognize Him? Do you know His name?"

"His name is Krishna." Everyone was stunned. It was Ann. Her disapproving, almost stern tone had a sobering effect. She had not appreciated their joking. Sanatan Swami nodded graciously and continued.

"Yes, His name is Krishna. I realize that it's difficult to accept the concept of a Supreme Personality, because our natural tendency is to think of Him as merely an extraordinary version of ourselves. To help us avoid making this common mistake Krishna explains in the *Bhagavad-gītā* the wonderful ways in which we can appreciate His manifestations in our own world. I'm thinking in particular of a few verses which give striking examples from nature. Krishna reveals what is called His 'universal form,' in which everything in the universe can at once be seen. Though advanced devotees are indeed more attached to Krishna's personal form, the universal form is especially meant for those whose spiritual vision is materialistic."

"Like us?" Winston asked. Sanatan Swami was amused. Winston was like a big child. "Not exactly, you're somewhere in between. But if you continue to take an interest, as you are now doing, you'll gradually understand. Ananta, why don't you read from the tenth chapter of the *Gītā*.

"Which verse should I begin from?" he asked, opening up the ancient text.

"Begin with the verse *aham ātmā guḍākeśa sarva-bhūtāśaya-sthitaḥ*."

Ananta began reading:

> I am the Supersoul, O Arjuna, seated in the hearts of all living entities. I am the beginning, the middle and the end of all beings.
>
> Of lights I am the radiant sun, and among the stars I am the moon.
>
> Of the senses I am the mind; and in living beings I am the living force [consciousness].
>
> Of bodies of water I am the ocean. And of immovable things I am the Himalayas.

"Are you beginning to understand? Although Krishna says that these manifestations are but a fragment of His potency, just see how grand they are. Please consider what this indicates about Krishna Himself, the Supreme Personality."

"That was beautiful!" Ann remarked. "Can we hear some more?"

> Of weapons I am the thunderbolt. Among subduers I am time, among beasts I am the lion. And of purifiers I am the wind.
>
> Of all sciences I am the spiritual science of the self. I am all-devouring death, and I am the generating principle of all that is yet to be.
>
> Of seasons I am flower-bearing spring. Of those who seek victory I am morality. Of secret things I am silence, and of the wise I am wisdom.
>
> Furthermore. O Arjuna, I am the generating seed of all existences. There is no being—moving or unmoving—that can exist without Me.

"It seems that everything in existence has some relationship to Krishna." Winston broke in. "What about us? What is our relationship with Krishna?"

Sanatan Swami's eyes brightened, but before he could respond Kuang Shi interjected, "Could we back up just a moment? Just before, you said that Krishna knows everything. How is He able to do that?"

"Because He's within the heart of all living beings, even within the atom," Sanatan Swami replied.

"You would have a hard time convincing scientists of that," said Kuang Shi.

"That's precisely the point—they aren't looking for Krishna in the heart of the atom, or anywhere for that matter. As Winston noted and as those verses we just cited emphasize, the point is to see the relationship between everything in nature and the Supreme Personality and ultimately the relationship between each of us and Krishna, the Supreme Personality of Godhead. Notice how Krishna says that He is represented by the lion among beasts or by the ocean among bodies of water. It's not that the ocean or the lion or the thunderbolt, say, is God, but that the best and finest of any mundane category you can think of represents the epitome of His potency in that field. So the simple question is, what human relationship represents the most sublime that one can have? The answer, of course, is a relationship with the Lord. If scientists don't want to be convinced of the interrelationship between Krishna and all aspects of creation, from the stars to atomic nuclei, then they'll just discover that material nature is. as Krishna says in *Bhagavad-gītā*, 'endlessly mutable,' *adhibhūtam kṣaro 'bhāvaḥ*."

It was Winston again who replied with a waggish, "Maharaj, you seemed to have answered both our questions at once." To which Sanatan Swami at once countered, "That's exactly the point, Winston. Any question you might have, whether about science, philosophy, or psychology, can be answered by the *Bhagavad-gītā*."

Kuang Shi spoke up, "Could you please explain more specifically how the individual and the Supreme are related? When we first met in the park you mentioned that the individual soul is located within each body. But just now you said that Krishna was in each body. I'm a little confused. Are they the same? Is the individual soul Krishna? Because what you've been saying about Krishna's manifestations in nature seems to indicate that they're different."

"The *Vedas* give a nice example to describe this dual phenomenon. The soul and the Supersoul, Krishna, are just like two birds in a tree. The individual soul is like a bird forever trying to enjoy the bitter fruits of the tree, while neglecting the sweet and loving relationship with his companion."

"But why does he go searching for all the bitter fruits, or whatever they are, and neglect the sweet relationship he has with his friend?" Kuang Shi inquired sincerely.

"Why, indeed." Sanatan Swami replied. "Doesn't make sense, does it? But the point is, we all do it. You should answer that question yourselves."

Each became thoughtful. "Is it because of ignorance?" Kuang Shi blurted out.

"Exactly! Due to ignorance we have forgotten our eternal relationship with Krishna." Sanatan Swami stood suddenly. "Come, I'll show you Krishna."

11

SANATAN SWAMI AND THE GROUP stood transfixed, while the two Deities stared back at them.

"You're looking at the worshipable Deities of Rādhā and Krishna."

"Lovely!" said Ann, voicing everyone's appreciation.

But Sanatan Swami knew they were appreciating what they considered to be mere statues. Yet they were intelligent and, given enough time, he was confident he could make them understand.

"When we accept Krishna as the Absolute Truth," he began, "we must also accept as absolute everything personally connected with Krishna: His name, His form, His qualities, His pastimes, His abode—all are Krishna. Now, I know what you're thinking, that the figures on the altar are just beautifully decorated marble statues. How could this possibly be God?"

"But they are made of marble. How can they be the Absolute Truth?" The question was Winston's, though it was certainly on all of their minds. "I mean, they are gorgeously outfitted—jewels, silk clothes, embroidered gowns, gold ornaments. It's fabulous! But ..."

Ann joined in: "Yes, they're so incredibly life-like. Look how Krishna is holding the flute; you can almost hear the notes. The way one leg is crossed over the other makes Him appear to be dancing. What did you say Her name is?" she asked, pointing to the Deity of Rādhā.

"Śrīmati Rādhārāni," Ananta said.

"She's so delicate and exquisite—especially that remarkable gown and the tiara She's wearing. My, She's so lovely. They seem so well matched."

"Yes, we think of Them as the perfection of all beauty," Sanatan Swami said.

"But Maharaj, I'm confused. They are beautiful, granted. That's one thing; we all appreciate the altar. But after all, They're still just statues. Why are you worshiping Them?"

"If He appeared in His form made of spiritual energy,

you wouldn't be able to see Him. Krishna is very merciful. He knows that as long as we are materially conditioned, we can see only matter. Therefore He appears before us in a form made of stone."

David pursued the point further. "But why this form? One could make any form one liked and worship it as the truth."

"Because the Deity conforms in every single detail—including the flute, tiara, in fact every feature you see here—to the descriptions found in eyewitness accounts of revealed scriptures. Many great sages, perfect in their spiritual vision, have confirmed that this is indeed a perfect likeness of Krishna. There are thousands of Krishna temples in India, and in every one of them Krishna looks the same. The worshipable form must therefore be authoritative.

"I'll give you an example. If you want to send a letter, what do you do? You either take it to the post office or drop it in a postal delivery box. If you think, 'Why should I bother to go to the post office? I'll make my own box and keep it in my apartment,' your letter will never be delivered, because the box that you have made is not authorized."

Kuang Shi asked, "Are there any similarities between the Krishna Deity you are worshiping here and the gods worshiped in the Chinese temples? The two forms of worship seem similar. The Chinese gods are also personal. They are dressed nicely, though certainly not so opulently, and they are served in a similar manner. They're also offered food, incense, and prayers, and people also bow down before them. Is there really any difference, or is it merely a question of choosing the right god to fulfill a particular desire?"

"Yes, in Chinese temples that I visited," began Sanatan Swami, "many varieties of deities are worshiped in order to fulfill particular desires. It is believed that if they are satisfied they can fulfill one's prayers. Thus the Chinese view their gods in a very pragmatic, almost materialistic way. One may pray to Krishna in the same way, but that is not considered pure devotional service. A pure devotee of Krishna tries to free himself of all material desires, realizing that as long as his material desires continue he will have to suffer the repetition of birth and death. He has only one prayer to Krishna: 'O Lord, please engage me in Your service.' That is the actual meaning of Hare Krishna, Hare Krishna, Krishna Krishna. Hare Hare / Hare Rama, Hare Rama, Rama Rama, Hare Hare. 'Hare' means 'the spiritual energy of the Lord,' personified in Srimati Radharani, whom you see here on your right," he added, pointing to the altar. " 'Krishna' and 'Rama' are names for the Supreme. Therefore, the Hare Krishna *mantra* is a prayer to Krishna to free us of our material desires."

Winston had studied the subject at school. "What you see here is called monotheism, or the worship of one absolute God. The Taoists on the other hand are polytheistic, worshiping many."

Red joined the discussion. "What would be your reply if someone said that Krishna is certainly in these statues, but He's also in the floor, the building, in us—in everything? Krishna is everything and everything is Krishna. What's your answer?"

"That's an excellent question, Red, and Krishna has dealt with it several times in the *Bhagavad-gītā*:

> The Supreme Personality of Godhead, who is greater than all, is attainable by unalloyed devotion. Although He is present in His abode. He is all-pervading, and everything is situated within Him.

"Krishna's being all-pervasive doesn't mean He has lost His individuality. He's present everywhere through His diverse energies. A businessman may sit in his office, but he is also present in each and every aspect of the business: his money, his factory, his equipment, and the workers who are answerable to him. At the same time, however, he remains an individual person apart from his business. This is only a material example, but it helps us understand Krishna's relationship with His unlimited potencies.

"So, Red, the answer to your question is that Krishna is everything, but nothing is Krishna save and except Krishna Himself—just as the businessman is everything in his business but nothing in the business equals the businessman. Is it clear?"

"Much more now, thanks."

"Yet there is a seeming philosophical paradox here—Krishna is and isn't present in the manifestations of His energy. This indicates that He can't be understood simply by logic alone or any sort of philosophical speculation. The only way the paradox can be resolved, Krishna says, is by devotional service to Him:

> To those who are constantly devoted to serving Me with love, I give the understanding by which they can come to Me.

"What you're saying, then, is that we should have blind faith," Red said deprecatingly.

"No, no! Never blind. Faith, yes, but not blind faith. At present our mind and senses are dulled, and we are unable to perceive Krishna. Unalloyed devotion means the process by which our senses become purified, and we are able to realize that when we stand before the Deities, as now, it is Krishna Himself whom we look upon. To begin the process, chanting the Hare Krishna *mantra* is most important. If you regularly practice the chanting on a daily basis, your faith will be confirmed by tangible experience."

Ann moved away from the small group to have a closer view of the Deities. "Who makes Their beautiful clothing?" she inquired. "Whoever it is must be very devoted to have taken such care. I've never seen such intricate hand-stitched embroidery. The flower garlands are absolutely beautiful!"

Sanatan Swami encouraged her. "Krishna is so merciful to come before us in this form to allow us to serve Him. Imagine if He were to be present only in His universal form—you remember, the form containing all the gigantic manifestations like the sun, moon, mountains, oceans, the wind? How could we possibly dress or feed Him? Could you imagine making a flower garland large enough? Because He is absolute. He is bigger than the biggest and smaller than the smallest—but here we see Him in His original, human-like feature, which is the most attractive. The next time you look through your telescope or microscope, try to find Him."

Everyone laughed. "I think it's easier and nicer to see Him here on the altar," Ann said.

"The more you think of Krishna—chanting His names, dressing Him, feeding Him—the less you'll be absorbed in your own bodily needs." Sanatan Swami looked at all of them and said with meaning, "That is the beginning of real loving devotion."

"Now, Maharaj, you're not suggesting we forgo all worldly pleasures, are you?" Winston's eyes grew wide, making the others laugh. "I mean, eating and dressing are just basic human needs."

Despite Winston's slightly humorous tone, it was a decent question. Sanatan Swami thought that they were willing enough to hear some philosophy about the Absolute Truth, but would they be equally receptive to learn the actual process of purification? Were they willing to sacrifice temporary material pleasures for ultimate spiritual benefits? He contemplated the best way to present the issue. "At present we are all covered by ignorance, thinking that we are our bodies. This body consciousness is not our original consciousness and it is the cause of all suffering. When we think only in terms of the body, we develop unlimited desires, and thus one is bound by a network of hopes and anxieties.

"To be free from ignorance we must become Krishna conscious, replacing our bodily-centered activities with activities centered around Krishna. Instead of thinking how to satisfy our appetite, think of how to satisfy Krishna's taste. Instead of thinking how to decorate our material bodies, which despite all our efforts grow old, become diseased, and die, let's think of decorating the beautiful forms of Radha and Krishna. The more you think of giving Krishna joy, the less you will be concerned with material sense enjoyment. I'm not suggesting that you deny your senses or your mind..."

"I hope not," Winston interjected.

Sanatan Swami continued, "At present the senses are in a diseased condition and they must be treated in order to cure them. When there is a disease in the eyes, the disease should be cured; plucking out the eyes is no treatment. Similarly, our material disease is based on the process of sense gratification, and to become cured from that diseased condition means to engage the senses in seeing the beauty of Krishna, hearing His glories, and always acting for His satisfaction. You see, Winston, I'm not recommending that the senses be denied."

"That's a very nice way of putting it," Kuang Shi said.

"In the *Bhagavad-gītā* Krishna explains that the senses will cease all material engagements only when they have a better activity to perform, just like the child who is mischievous cannot be stopped unless given better play. Then automatically he will stop his mischievousness. In the same way, the improper activities of our senses can be stopped only by better engagement in relationship with the Supreme Person, Krishna. And when you forget sense gratification entirely, then you are qualified for returning back to Godhead."

"Back to Godhead? Where's that?" David asked.

"Beyond this solar system and beyond this universe. The spiritual world is described in *Bhagavad-gītā*. It is eternal and transcendental to this material manifestation. When this world ceases to exist, the spiritual world with its unlimited spiritual planets will remain unaffected. It is the destination for those who become Krishna conscious. When a devotee returns there, he never comes back to take birth again in this material world. That's what going 'back to Godhead' means."

They were eager to hear more about this spiritual world. "Planets in the spiritual world are made of spiritual energy and are self-effulgent. There is no need of illumination from a sun, or a moon, or electricity. This is the supreme abode of Lord Krishna, where all desires are fulfilled. It is known as Vrindavan and is full of palaces made of spiritual gems. There are also trees called desire trees, which can supply any type of food you desire ..."

"Take me there! Take me there!" Winston feigned.

"... and there are cows known as surabhi cows, which supply unlimited milk. Krishna is served by hundreds and thousands of devotees. He is known as Govinda, just as our Deity here in New York is named Radha-Govinda. There's no equal to His beauty and attractiveness. The pure devotees of Krishna always desire His association, and sometimes, just to please them, Krishna descends within this world."

"The same Krishna?" Winston asked.

"What happens to the spiritual world when Krishna leaves to come here?" David asked, puzzled.

"Excellent question, and the answer is that nothing changes, because Krishna is unlimited. He can be simultaneously present in all places at once. You or I obviously cannot do this, but neither are we supreme and absolute. There is no difficulty, however, for Krishna to expand Himself unlimitedly. Whenever Krishna comes within the material world at His scheduled time. He restores the principles of religion and satisfies His pure devotees in all respects."

One particular point fascinated Kuang Shi, and he asked for clarification. "When Krishna comes, does He have a material body like ours? Also, what did you mean when you said that He comes according to a particular schedule?"

"When Krishna descends. He doesn't have to change bodies as we do. He comes in His original spiritual form, and therefore His body is not subject to old age, disease, or death. For example, there's no picture of Krishna with grey hair or a beard, although He had children, grandchildren, and great-grandchildren."

"Krishna had children?" The question came from Mary.

"Yes, why not? The Absolute Truth is complete in all respects. If mortals can have children, why not the Supreme Absolute Truth? But His children are not ordinary, nor are any of the others who associate with Him. Just as Krishna comes in His original form, so also do His eternal associates, many of whom accompany Him from the spiritual world when He comes here. Even in ordinary affairs, an important person never travels alone. Getting back to Kuang Shi's question ..."

"Wait!" Mary interrupted. "I want to ask more questions about Krishna's family."

"Let me answer Kuang Shi's question first. There are as

many incarnations of Krishna as there are waves in the ocean. In other words, the number is unlimited. The scheduling of His personal appearance is calculated as follows: The universe exists for three hundred eleven trillion and forty million earth years. This is equal to one hundred years on the highest planet, known in Sanskrit as Brahmaloka. Calculating time according to that planet, Krishna comes once in a day of Brahma, who is the secondary creator of the material universe. The last time He appeared in this universe was approximately five thousand years ago, and He stayed for one hundred twenty-five years. His activities are recorded in a book known as the *Śrīmad-Bhāgavatam*.

"Krishna appeared most recently only five hundred years ago. Realizing that the principles of religion were deteriorating rapidly in this age. He saw the need to propagate a spiritual practice strong enough to counteract the anomalies of this age. Thus He came as Lord Chaitanya and taught the chanting of the holy names: Hare Krishna, Hare Krishna, Krishna Krishna, Hare Hare / Hare Rama, Hare Rama, Rama Rama, Hare Hare. As Lord Chaitanya, Krishna disguised Himself as a devotee in order to teach others by His own example. Lord Chaitanya experienced the highest ecstasy through dancing and chanting the glories of the holy name. And traveling throughout India, He induced this same devotional fervor. Whoever had His association, even for a moment, became overwhelmed with divine love."

At that moment the sound of loudly beating drums caught everyone's attention, and they all turned. A large crowd had gathered at the opposite end of the temple room, near the shrine of the founder.

"What is it?" asked Ann.

"Some ceremony, I guess," Winston said. They all

strained to see.

Sanatan Swami explained. "This ceremony is called *kirtan*. Everyone is expected to join in." Without saying anything further, he took Winston and Kuang Shi by the hand, the others following behind, and led them into the large crowd, which numbered well over a thousand persons.

The drummers were ready, more than twenty of them. The drums were cylindrical and had straps to enable them to be hung around the neck, thus allowing the drummers to dance too. In addition to the drummers, at least one hundred persons played hand cymbals, which they beat in time with the rhythm of the drums. The musicians divided themselves into six groups, four drums and sixteen sets of cymbals in each. They spread out to occupy the entire temple room. Each group had two lead singers and four lead dancers.

When all parties were properly aligned, the lead singers began to sing in unison Hare Krishna, Hare Krishna, Krishna Krishna, Hare Hare / Hare Rama, Hare Rama, Rama Rama, Hare Hare. Responding to their lead the cymbals and drums took up the rhythm and began to play. The response from the more than one thousand assembled devotees was deafening. One thousand voices sang in unison, uplifting everyone's spirit. Everyone in the hall chanted, and as the rhythmic beats picked up momentum, the whole assembly danced.

The lead dancers in each group had their followers dance in step, each swaying backward and forward, their hands held aloft. They danced in a circle, and as the tempo increased they began to spin and jump in the air, their faces beaded with perspiration.

Inspired by their dancing, the drummers played intricate beats on their two-headed drums, and the measured beats further enlivened the dancers and singers. The hundred pairs of cymbals chimed in time, their clear, bell-like tones creating a celestial sound.

The thousand-strong chorus sang from their hearts with devotional fervor, a great symphony of human voices. Their powerful singing rent the air, shook the windows, and drove away every thought except, Krishna, Krishna, Krishna, from the hearts of all. Hare Krishna, Hare Krishna, Krishna Krishna, Hare Hare / Hare Rama, Hare Rama, Rama Rama, Hare Hare. Nothing else was spoken, nothing else heard, no other thought pondered.

Kuang Shi was deeply affected by the exuberance of it all. It seemed to him that the holy names of Krishna were melting his heart and driving away all doubts from his mind. The Absolute Truth had descended in transcendental sound. Winston was deluged by a mercy that swept away all his misgivings in a flood of happiness.

Ananta looked at their blissful faces, Ann's eyes in particular, sparkling with joyful tears. They all seemed to radiate a great love, elevated by their spiritual vision. If only this consciousness could always be maintained, Ananta thought, there would be no envy, no anger, nor malice.

For more than an hour the chanting continued to soar, lifting them all to heights of spiritual ecstasy.

12

KUANG SHI PUSHED HIS CHAIR away from the electron microscope and went over to the window to watch the rain beating upon the cement sidewalk below. He had been alone all afternoon, but he was not fully concentrating on the work at hand. Other thoughts occupied his mind.

He looked down at the wet sidewalk, then out across the grounds separating the medical wing from the rest of the building. For a moment he felt as though he were in Beijing. He imagined himself standing in a similar laboratory in the People's Liberation Army General Hospital. The weather could easily have been the same. In fact, it might have been the weather that pulled his thoughts halfway around the world.

No, it wasn't that. It was the meeting of the government representative Dr. Zhang Chong Shu echoing in his mind. "Has Li Kuang Shi no love for his country? Has he no feeling for its honor? Has he forgotten its people?"

How could he ever forget? He remembered, yes, but the memories were bitter-sweet, yet he doubted that he would ever feel wholly at home amongst the people here. He had left all his friends and family—he choked, remembering his father and mother, whom he had not seen for years. He swallowed hard, his eyes moist. There were new friends now. His uncle and aunt had been kind to him, but who could ever replace his father and mother? And what were all his old friends doing now?

No, he could never forget them. Nor could he forget the Chinese nation, of which he was a part. His people had struggled under the weight of feudalism for so many centuries. Now at last they were liberated. A new nation, hardly forty years old, looking ahead to a bright future. Was there a Chinese who did not want to be part of that future?

Kuang Shi turned from the window and faced the enameled row of shelves holding their labeled bottles, the steel tables and equipment, and as he did so the voice of China seemed to drift away. Yes, he was making a sacrifice, but it was not due to selfishness. If he was going to serve mankind, then America was the best place to do it. Or was it?

Again he turned and looked out the window. His government had made an attractive offer: a fully-equipped research department in a leading hospital, and he the chief of research, the one who would determine the direction of the work. Until Dr. Zhang's visit, he had more or less resolved to accept a position that had opened in the National Institute of Allergy and Infectious Diseases located in Bethesda. Maryland. But he would only be one of many assistants, and he would be lucky if they allowed him to specialize in the field of his interest. Besides, he knew only too well the prejudice that existed against those who were not Americans by birth. Of course, he would have the best of up-to-date equipment at his disposal. But would he be allowed to do the work he wanted? This was the big question. The salary did not concern him. If it was money he was after, he would have accepted the offers of Abbott Laboratories or Hoffmann-La Roche, either of which would have paid three times what he would make with the National Institute.

His stream of thoughts was suddenly interrupted.

"Charles, are you busy?" Ann leaned in the door, only her head and the white smock covering her street clothes visible. Kuang Shi invited her in.

"I haven't been able to concentrate on my work today," she said.

"Neither have I," admitted Kuang Shi.

"Hare Krishna!" she said with a big smile.

"What? Oh!" Kuang Shi suddenly caught on. "Hare Krishna."

"I can't get the chanting off my mind."

"It is infectious," Kuang Shi agreed. "I've been chanting on the beads Ananta gave us, and I've been completing four times around the beads each day. What about you?"

Ann did not want to appear as excited as she actually felt. "I started like you, with four. But last evening I just felt like I could chant all night. I actually completed sixteen rounds. Charles, it was a wonderful experience!"

Kuang Shi looked at Ann closely. He knew her well enough to see that she was feeling a genuine attachment to the chanting. She had often displayed such enthusiasm, but it was always for her research work. This was the first time he could remember her sharing with him such a personal experience.

"How does the chanting make you feel, Charles?"

Kuang Shi thought for a moment. "Calm." He paused. "Free from worries. A kind of inner satisfaction. Something like the way I feel when I've completed a really productive day in the lab." He shrugged his shoulders. "It's really hard to describe."

"I like chanting individually with the beads. But it's hard to equal the experience when we all chanted together on Sunday. I don't think I'll ever forget that feeling." She hopped up on the high stool and swiveled about a full three hundred sixty degrees. "What's your impression of Sanatan Swami?"

From the way she asked the question, Kuang Shi could sense her feelings. At that moment he realized that he had not actually revealed to anyone else what his real feelings were. "What he's taught me has made a deep impression," he began. "At first, my mind fought with nearly everything he said. But it's hard to defeat the logic. He's so clear-headed and vastly learned. After a while I just stopped trying."

"Do you sometimes feel that he can read your mind? I mean, understand your deepest thoughts?" She didn't wait for his reply. "I feel as though he knows me much better than I know myself. And I feel as though he cares about me more than anyone ever has." There was silence. "Maybe I'm just being sentimental," she added, embarrassed for having revealed her inner feelings.

"I think I understand." Kuang Shi said after some time.

"He reminds me of my father."

"Charles, there's something I want to tell you that I haven't told anyone. I think you'll understand."

Kuang Shi wondered what it was. He couldn't imagine that there was something that Ann would tell him and not her parents, or David.

"When you first invited the Swami to meet us here at Columbia, it wasn't my first contact with Krishna consciousness. You see, one of my best friends—you remember Lisa?" Kuang Shi shook his head negatively. "... anyway, she used to go to Columbia but transferred to the University of California at Berkeley. She's become deeply involved with Krishna consciousness and she's been sending me some books. I didn't take it seriously at first, until one day she sent me *Easy Journey to Other Planets*."

"The same book sparked my interest also," he said excitedly, remembering when Ananta first gave it to him.

Ann continued, "That book really started me thinking. We've always been taught that life could be explained by chemical evolution. You know, the primordial chemical soup, the big bang? It started me thinking, and I began to realize that when it comes to issues like these, science is simply bluffing." Kuang Shi smiled. She hopped down from her chair. "So you think I'm deluding myself? You think I'm becoming just a superstitious fool?" Actually Kuang Shi didn't think any of these things—he agreed with her. But she was too excited for him to get a word in. "Well, Dr. Li, let me remind you that I am also a scientist. I can give you scientific proof that we scientists, as a group, are a big bluff!"

Kuang Shi held his hand up and laughed. "Stop! Stop! Ann, I agree with you. Naturally I haven't admitted it to anyone because they'd probably think I was crazy." Ann was visibly amazed. "I mean, I don't have all the answers," Kuang Shi continued, "but it's obvious that there are so many questions which science cannot yet answer and in all likelihood they'd never be able to answer fully."

"But they won't admit it!" Ann said angrily. "They've been accepted as authorities by everyone and they've become so attached to the—" she searched for the right word "—worship! I just read one book about the origin and nature of life by a Nobel Prize winner. You know, Francis Crick?" Naturally Kuang Shi knew the name. Crick and his associate Watson were the co-discoverers of DNA.

Ann fished around in her handbag and pulled out a small pocket book. "Here it is. Listen to how he starts the book: There is one fact about the origin of life which is reasonably certain. Whenever and wherever it happened, it started a very long time ago, so long ago that it is extremely difficult to form any realistic idea of such vast stretches of time.'"

"If it's so difficult to have any realistic idea, then what is he writing about?" Kuang Shi remarked.

"Charles, you won't believe the next quote: 'An honest man, armed with all the knowledge available to us now, could only state that in some sense, the origin of life appears at the moment to be almost a miracle, so many are the conditions which would have to have been satisfied to get it going.' This is the so-called scientific statement of a Nobel Laureate. Why it's something you'd expect a religious person to say, not a scientist."

"I've read the book," Kuang Shi said. "He admits he can't unravel the mystery of life, and so instead he comes up with this theory of 'Directed Panspermia'! Can you believe it! A civilization from a distant universe sent a rocket full of microorganisms to be released in earth's atmosphere in order to generate life here."

"And where did that higher civilization come from?" Ann demanded.

"That he doesn't say."

"He takes such great pains to deny any possibility of there being a supreme intelligent being who created life, yet he expects us to accept his suggestion that life was sent here by some higher civilization. What's the difference?!"

"None at all." Kuang Shi said. "If one's not possible, how could the other one be?"

"I think I understand why scientists like Crick think that religious beliefs are outmoded. I shared the same thoughts myself. I was raised a Christian, but I realized that their beliefs didn't coincide with scientific facts, so I lost all my interest in religion. It disturbed my family members and friends a lot, but what was I to do? You probably never faced such problems in China, since atheism is more or less an official part of the philosophy." Even were it not, Kuang Shi thought, Chinese people would never argue with their elders the way Americans do. He continued to listen. "When I started reading the Vedic literatures, I found them very different from all other scriptures I had studied. Krishna consciousness is not only reasonable, it's scientific! If Crick and other scientists would just study the *Vedas*, they could find so much information that they are looking for. But they're always under the impression that all the great achievements in world history have been produced by Western civilization."

"Western civilization is fairly recent compared with the ancient civilization of China," said Kuang Shi proudly.

"China, and India too. Sanatan Swami says that the *Vedas* have been around for thousands of years. I'm convinced that civilization isn't a matter of skyscraper buildings and jet planes. You know, Charles, what it really comes down to is spiritualism versus materialism."

Kuang Shi poured them each a glass of water. Ann sipped hers slowly. "Well, now you know my inner thoughts," she said. "But there's one thing more. I've reached an important decision. You remember Śrīla

Prabhupāda, the founder of the Krishna movement? He said that if any scientists were convinced of the veracity of Krishna consciousness, then they should utilize their knowledge to establish the principle that life comes from life, not from chemicals. Charles! He wants us to prove scientifically that Krishna is the source of all life." Ann paused for a moment to reflect. "He asked for the construction of a model of the universe based on Vedic descriptions. A group of Krishna conscious scientists have formed the Bhaktivedanta Institute to do this." She paused for effect. "I'm thinking about working with them."

"Would you be giving up your career?" Kuang Shi asked.

"Of course not! The Institute is an international fellowship, so I can participate without having to stop my research. There's one more thing, Charles. I've decided to start following the principles of Krishna consciousness." She paused. "I've been thinking about it for some time, but it was the chanting that convinced me it's the right thing to do." Kuang Shi had no immediate reply. "Charles, I've got to finish up in the lab and get home. Can we talk some more about this tomorrow?" As she turned to leave, she looked back at Kuang Shi. "Hare Krishna, Charles."

"Hare Krishna, Ann."

Kuang Shi returned to the window. It was still raining. Americans are so different from the Chinese, Kuang Shi thought. Ann was typically strong-willed and independent, a real individualist. That was the main difference, individualism. A Chinese person would never behave so independently. First, he'd consult his parents and other close family members. But for Americans, family meant husband, wife, and children: elders were seldom, if ever, consulted.

Still, each culture had personality traits not easily changed. Americans seemed to derive strength by asserting their individuality, whereas Chinese preferred the security of a group. But all this could quickly change. Confucianism had emphasized obedience as opposed to independence. Kuang Shi thought they both had value. He hoped that in their efforts to improve, the Chinese people would not have to sacrifice the advantages of either.

Returning to her apartment, Ann found the front door unlocked. She was certain she had locked it.

"Anyone here?" she called out a bit fearfully.

"It's me, Ann." She was relieved to hear David's voice.

"David! I thought you had gone to Connecticut this morning." She went first to the kitchen and unpacked the groceries and then poured a little milk into a dish for her cat.

"Ann, just what are you doing?" David sounded a bit impatient.

"I'm just feeding the cat and watering the plants. I'll be there in a second." She hung up her coat and came into the sitting room. "Well, what kept you back?" David wasn't sitting in his favorite rocker. Reclined on the sofa, he looked sullen. When he pouted like this, she thought, he was like a small child. She went about the room watering each of the plants. "Well, what's wrong?"

David continued to sulk, remaining silent.

She tried to enliven him. "Okay. Let me guess. Your mother phoned to tell you your uncle Harry is visiting and you don't want to see him? The blueprints for your townhouse design were rejected? Your liver is acting up again?"

"What makes you so damned cheerful?" he glowered.

"And why shouldn't I be cheerful?" She smiled bright-faced as she began to rock in the large wooden rocker.

David sat up. "You've been acting strange these past few days."

"I have not."

David studied her. "Somehow, you seem different," he said irascibly.

"I'm the same Ann Denton: five foot six inches, black hair, brown eyes, and ready to fight at the drop of a hat. So be careful."

"That's not what I meant."

"Well, what do you mean?" she stopped rocking.

"I mean, ever since Sunday, you've been avoiding me."

Ann smiled. David had a special way of endearing himself.

"Well, with so many infectious diseases spreading everywhere, I was just trying to be careful," she joked. In fact, she had been keeping aloof in order to reach some important decisions.

She got up and walked over to where David was sitting, and, giving him a light kiss on the forehead, sat down next to him. "See! I'm as sweet as always."

"I'm not impressed." he said coolly. He got up and began to pace.

Ann wondered what to do. David knew her all too well. It was difficult to keep anything from him for long. And what was the point? She had had enough time to think things over and knew what she wanted.

"Well, maybe I have been a little distant. I needed the space to think things out and gather my thoughts."

"To think what out?" David had stopped pacing and stood directly before her.

Ann hesitated. "About the direction of my life."

"And just what does that mean?" he demanded, though he already suspected.

"I'm joining the Red Cross to do relief work in Ethiopia."

"Stop joking!"

There was no point to holding back. He was just becoming more irritable. "Alright, I'll tell you. I've decided to be a Krishna devotee."

"I thought so! But you're a scientist ..."

"I'm being as methodical as always."

"But you just met those Krishna people a week ago. What do you know about their philosophy? I mean, I heard the guy speak just like you did, and..."

"... He's not a 'guy,'" Ann snapped. "If you're going to be disrespectful, I'd rather not continue."

David was getting a little worried. "You're really serious about this, aren't you? Alright. I heard everything the Swami said. He's a pretty impressive guy, but as a way of life, forget it!"

"David, if we're going to talk about this sensibly, then at least sit down." Grudgingly he sat in the rocker. Ann looked at him. This was the man whom she would one day marry. It was essential that she try to make him understand. "I didn't just begin to learn about Krishna a week ago. I've been studying their books for nearly three years." She paused. David looked shocked, almost betrayed. She hoped he would understand. "You remember my friend Lisa?" David nodded, stunned. "She's been regularly sending me books ever since she moved to California, and I've been reading them, though I've never mentioned anything to anyone."

"But you've never discussed anything with me." David felt deceived.

"It was something I wasn't sure about. It was so different from anything I'd ever read. I wasn't certain what others might think. I mean, our families are all Christians. And the biochem people are mostly atheists. So I just kept everything to myself, reading and trying to understand the philosophy better. It makes so much sense. I sometimes wonder why everyone doesn't accept it. David, I want to be able to discuss this with you. It would be such a relief. We've never had any secrets from each other."

David listened with stony silence, but Ann went on. "I think people will gradually accept Krishna consciousness more and more. Ananta was explaining to me—you remember, Ananta was the young disciple of Sanatan Swami—he was explaining to me that more than one third of all Americans accept reincarnation as a fact and nearly five percent are following a vegetarian diet in part. To have influenced such a large number of people within only twenty years is quite an accomplishment, don't you think?"

David was thinking of many things. He didn't know where to begin. "You want to be a vegetarian?" he said almost in disbelief. It was one of many questions spinning in his mind.

"Vegetarians are healthier, they live longer. I'll get a cookbook for us. One of the Krishna women just published a cookbook that was voted the book of the year. You loved the dinner we had at the temple on Sunday, remember? You said it was the best feast you ever had." She paused. "Another thing is. I'm not going to drink wine anymore."

"No wine?"

"No intoxication of any kind. I'm going to purify myself." David felt ill. It was as if someone had kicked him in the stomach. Worse, as if he had suddenly received the news of the death of someone very close. His face lost color.

"Anything else?" It was all that he could manage to ask.

"Well, the next thing is a little more difficult." She hesitated, holding her breath. "We shouldn't sleep together until after we're married."

"That's ridiculous'." David exploded.

"And when we do, it should be for having a child," she added.

He was furious. "Not for fun, right?" This was turning into a nightmare. He wished he could wake up and end it. Unfortunately, it wasn't that easy. What's she thinking of? What would others think?

"Have you told anyone else about these ideas?"

"Only Charles."

"And what does he think?"

"He found it quite reasonable."

"Of course he did! He's not going to be your husband like I am!"

"David, be reasonable."

"It's you who's not being reasonable. Do you call reasonable to feed your husband a plate of raw vegetables every night? Is it reasonable for a man not to want to make love to his wife? It's not only reasonable, it's natural! I don't want to marry a nun!" He was fuming. There was no use arguing further. He grabbed his jacket and walked out, slamming the door behind him.

Ann sat quietly alone with only David's anger to keep her company. She went over the conversation in her mind, wondering if she had made a mistake. No matter what she might have said, it would have infuriated him. He was jealous, but jealous of whom? Krishna? But that was silly. She wouldn't love him any less. In fact, more.

It was better to let him cool down. He would walk for an hour or two and then come back. Then she would reassure him of her feelings for him, speak sweetly, and let him understand that her feelings for him had not changed at all.

She searched her handbag, reaching for the chanting beads. She began to chant softly to herself: Hare Krishna,

Hare Krishna, Krishna Krishna, Hare Hare/ Hare Rama, Hare Rama, Rama Rama, Hare Hare.

David went directly to Kuang Shi's room. He knocked strongly on the door.

When Kuang Shi heard David's voice, he immediately let him in. It was clear that David was upset.

"David, is something wrong?"

"Can we sit down?" David's mood lacked his usual politeness. He was flushed. They sat facing each other.

David came immediately to the point. "This Krishna thing has gone too far. Ann told me she spoke with you. If you want to ruin your life, that's your business, but don't interfere with mine." It was hard to imagine David saying such things.

"There must be some misunderstanding..."

David cut him off. "I'm not interested in any Eastern way of life. I was born an American and that's what I want to stay."

"David, calm down!" Kuang Shi said strongly. "Let me get you some water." David wasn't interested. "There's a misunderstanding. Ann's come to her decisions on her own. I never influenced her in any way."

"I'm sorry for blaming you, Charles. I should have known better. But she's suggesting a complete change of lifestyle, and I'm not going along with it."

"From what I've understood of the Krishna philosophy," Kuang Shi said, "it's neither Eastern nor Western. It deals with the soul and the Supreme Soul, nothing material. Maybe you'll have to adjust your life a little, but I don't think it will mean anything extreme. Perhaps you should find out more about it before coming to any hasty conclusions. Ann mentioned to me that she had studied the literature for three years. She's a very intelligent woman and I've never known her to make many mistakes."

David composed himself. "I guess it was all so different, I became too alarmed. Still, I think that she's gone too far too quickly. She listens to you, Charles. She respects you incredibly. She's told me that many times. Won't you speak to her? Advise her to be a bit more considerate; not just for my sake, but for all those close to her. You know we're planning to get married. I don't want those plans to be disturbed by something like this. Please talk to her."

"I'll do my best," Kuang Shi promised.

"I was supposed to visit my parents the rest of the week. I think I'll go now. It'll give me time to think about everything. In the meantime, I hope you do speak to her."

Kuang Shi had an inspiration. He reached for his copy of the *Bhagavad-gītā*. "David, why don't you take this with you. It may help you to have a better idea of how Ann is actually thinking." David didn't refuse. Feeling embarrassed, he excused himself again and took his leave.

13

KUANG SHI, ANN, AND WINSTON surfaced from the subway station and came out upon the imposing statue of Christopher Columbus. Kuang Shi smiled at how much had taken place in the few weeks since he had last been here. This is where he had met Ananta for the first time. That had also been a Friday evening, and once again he was to meet Ananta.

From a distance came the faint but distinct sound of drums and cymbals. Ananta had assured them that congregational street chanting was even more ecstatic than what they had experienced at the temple the previous Sunday. They were excited. Krishna consciousness was exciting. To apply the teachings to one's life was challenging, yet the more one surrendered the more Krishna enabled one to overcome the challenges. It was a philosophy that could be fully appreciated only by practice, and they felt good about the progress they had made during the week. Like school children eager to bring their homework to their teacher for approval, they looked forward to meeting Sanatan Swami. They hoped he would recognize in their blissful faces the effects of his teaching. They had no doubt in his ability to teach and were quickly gaining confidence in their ability to learn. It was as if Krishna were inspiring them from within.

While riding the subway they had chanted on their beads, attracting many curious looks from fellow passengers. Some young people had even come over and inquired from them, and Winston had explained the purpose of chanting. Identifying oneself with Krishna gave anyone who was interested an opportunity to find out what you were doing. That little taste of preaching whetted their appetites for the big festival they were about to join.

As the drums and cymbals grew stronger in volume and the chanting grew clearly audible, their eagerness increased. At every moment they expected to see the devotees. They turned the corner at Broadway, and wave upon wave of jubilant devotees surged toward them with thunderous sounds. Suddenly they were engulfed, swept up in the ocean of sound. Like deep-sea swimmers, they bobbed up and down, sometimes floating, sometimes submerged in the waves of the holy names: Hare Krishna, Hare Krishna, Krishna Krishna, Hare Hare / Hare Rama, Hare Rama, Rama Rama, Hare Hare.

The procession of over two hundred covered the broad sidewalk of New York's busiest street like a massive tidal wave, sweeping all up in its path. Shoppers, workers, businessmen, officials, tourists—everyone—were inundated by the holy names of Krishna. Some tried to take shelter in nearby shops, others dodged traffic to cross to the other side, but no one could avoid the flood of mercy as it crashed against buildings, swirled about automobiles, and sprayed the faces of an astonished multitude.

The chanters laughed and leaped high, feeling unbounded bliss as they eagerly drank the nectar of the sound of the holy names, wishing that they had hundreds of tongues and thousands of ears to relish the sweet sounds of the Hare Krishna *mantra*.

From street to street the wave moved, heading south like a great army. Visitors to New York City wondered what it was, but before they could get an answer they were deafened by the chanting, which resounded between the buildings and reverberated to the sky. Yet thousands got their answers that night in the wake of the storm that left them each holding a transcendental book to tell them they had just witnessed the eternal celebration of the congregational chanting of the Lord's holy name.

Krishna, the Supreme Controller of man's destinies, directs the wanderings of all living beings. Certainly, then. Krishna must have had a special purpose in mind when He arranged for Lawrence Chung and his wife Shiao Lin to be present among the hundreds of thousands who witnessed the chanting. And just as surely it must have been Krishna who directed Lawrence Chung's vision to see among the hundreds of chanters his nephew Li Kuang Shi.

The two stared, mouths agape, too shocked to speak. At last Lawrence turned to his wife, horrified.

"Shiao Lin, it's our Charlie!"

"My sister's son!" she cried out.

The image of their nephew dancing wildly in public, his arms flailing high in the air, screaming at the top of his lungs impressed itself indelibly on their minds. Charlie Li! Dr. Li! A Hare Krishna?! Never! Never so long they lived!

14

NI DONGBUDONG? Chung Shiao Lin stared irritably at Kuang Shi. Why was her nephew being so stubborn? Couldn't he see what a perfect arrangement it was?

Mrs. Yang Po Ling was fidgeting uncomfortably. Both she and her daughter Carolyn felt extremely embarrassed. Why, she wondered, was Shiao Lin so insistent? She would never have agreed to the meeting except for Shiao Lin's certainty. Shiao Lin had as much as told her that her nephew was eager to be engaged to her daughter. Within minutes the boy's hesitancy was obvious, but Shiao Lin had been carrying on for nearly half an hour!

Lawrence Chung sat strangely silent. He had barely uttered a word the whole time. It was a crazy idea, as far as he was concerned. The last thing young people wanted these days was to have some bossy relatives telling them whom to marry. He looked at his two kids, Johnny and Susan, casually sprawled out on the carpet reading the Sunday newspapers. He could see that they were amused by the whole thing, and educated as well. They'd never let their parents do this to them. Lawrence decided to let it go for a few more minutes and then end it.

Shiao Lin was exasperated. What more could she say? Her unfailing sense of duty made her indifferent to everyone else's growing impatience. She would try again.

"Kuang Shi, be sensible!" she urged. "You will never find a better wife than Carolyn. Her mother has trained her perfectly at home, she's well organized, an excellent cook, frugal, and never loses her temper. She's highly educated and as beautiful as a lotus."

"Mrs. Chung, please!" Carolyn protested. But Shiao Lin wasn't listening. Ever since Kuang Shi had arrived from China, she had looked after him like a mother. With his parents thousands of miles away there was no one else to protect him. And they were depending on her. Time and time again his mother had written her that she should look after him like her own son. And Shiao Lin had given her word, taking the request to heart. So now she had to save him. Yes, save him from becoming a monk! It would be worse than suicide!

Marriage was the answer. "It is a match made in heaven. You are highly educated, a scientist, strong, healthy, even-tempered. And she is equally qualified. Our two families are known to each other for such a long time. Your mother has written me that this will be a perfect marriage."

Kuang Shi sat between his aunt and uncle, his mind in a quandary. He respected them no less than he did his own parents. There was no way to estimate how much they had helped him, nor had he any doubt of their good intentions in trying to arrange this marriage. He could not remember a time when he had disregarded any of their advice. Their experience in worldly affairs was far more than his, and their predictions had invariably proved true. But the present issue was a real dilemma. He could easily appreciate Carolyn's good qualities. In fact, were he to marry, it would be a woman like her. The problem was not Carolyn, nor ultimately the idea of marriage. It was much more complex than that.

The last few weeks of intensive association with the devotees had caused him to contemplate the purpose of his life now more than ever before and to put aside his personal interests to consider the welfare of his fellow humans. He saw the visit of the Chinese government's representative as some special sign—was it Krishna? Dr. Zhang's offer seemed the most likely way to fulfill his desire.

There was a maze of issues to consider, not the least of which was the present request being made him. By

Yoga for the New Millennium 153

accepting his aunt's proposal he would at least in some way fulfill his indebtedness to them, but his engagement to Carolyn would have to go on for several years, at least until he was properly situated. More significantly, would they be able to appreciate his desire to return to China?

The pleading voice of his aunt penetrated his thoughts, forcing him to choose. Though full of uncertainty, he uttered, "Alright!"

"Alright?" repeated his uncle questioningly. "Did you say 'alright'?" But there was no doubt what he had said, and all had heard him clearly. There was no ending to their joy. His cousin Susan leaped up clapping and ran to Carolyn, embracing her. Mrs. Yang and his aunt and uncle were shaking hands excitedly. Johnny looked up from the sports page and grinned.

Kuang Shi's mind was racing. He had agreed, but there were conditions.

"Wait!" he said, barely noticed by the others. They had nearly forgotten him in their excitement. "Wait!" he repeated, this time much more loudly. That got their attention, and they waited expectantly.

They were all smiles now. Kuang Shi also started to laugh, and as he began to talk his words became tangled. "I want to explain a few things," he began. They sat down, controlling their happiness, expecting some sort of felicitous speech.

"I've agreed, of course"—he looked especially at Carolyn and Mrs. Yang. "But you should understand why I took so long to decide. I was thinking of my career, because that's most important to me. Of course, I was also thinking of all of you. You are very important to me too. I chose to be a scientist because of my interest in helping others. My father always taught me not to be selfish, but to put others' interests first."

"That's very noble, Charles, very noble of you," Mrs. Yang said admiringly to her future son-in-law.

"Therefore I hope you'll understand that everything must take secondary importance to my work." Aunt Shiao Lin agreed that this was quite reasonable. "I hope you'll therefore appreciate that when I agreed to be engaged to Carolyn," he smiled looking at her, "I was not thinking that we would get married immediately."

"Certainly not, certainly not," Mrs. Yang confirmed. "A proper time of waiting should be there."

"Yes, and I was thinking that a proper time would be three or four years." The words had hardly come out of Kuang Shi's mouth, when there was a barrage of protest from everyone in the room. Carolyn looked especially vexed. Mrs. Yang tried to show her as much sympathy as possible without offending her future son-in-law. When the commotion had subsided, Kuang Shi continued. "Recently I have received a very attractive offer that will allow me to concentrate fully on my field. I've been offered the position of chief of research at a major hospital with full government funding."

"Why, that's wonderful, Charles!" Mrs. Yang exclaimed.

"Where? Which hospital?" Uncle Lawrence asked, a little less enthusiastically.

Kuang Shi calmly announced, "The People's Liberation Army General Hospital." It was as if he had thrown a bomb in their midst.

Above the commotion Lawrence Chung was most vociferous. "You must be crazy! Go back to China?! For what?"

"To serve my country."

"Charlie, listen to me. Have I ever misled you?" Kuang Shi shook his head silently. "This Chinese government will make so many promises which they'll never fulfill. It happens all the time. They're poor, Charlie. They're losing their best students. They're desperate. They'll promise you anything, and when you go there you'll be at their mercy."

"But Dr. Zhang Chong Shu seemed very genuine. He's the president of a respected scientific association. He was formerly a member of the World Health Organization in Switzerland. Men like him don't have to lie."

Lawrence Chung was distraught. "Charlie, you don't know. Don't I always tell you how naive you are? Politicians always lie. It's part of their job."

Shiao Lin spoke up. "Do we have to remind you how much the Chinese people suffered in the last forty years? Do we have to remind you how they practically destroyed our country during the Cultural Revolution?"

"But times have changed. It's not like that anymore. A new China is being built now. They want young leaders, men like myself. They're not afraid to admit their wrongs. Why should I deny them?"

"How can you deny us? And after all these years!" Lawrence Chung reached across his nephew, placing his hand on his wife's shoulder. "Look at your aunt, look at her! She's crying. Do you know how this is hurting her? She loves you like a son and you're putting a knife into her heart!" Kuang Shi almost cried, but he held back the tears, his heart stung by the pain of his uncle's words.

The atmosphere was somber and tense. At last Mrs. Yang spoke. "We are all very shocked, Charles. Shocked and disappointed. You didn't even bother to confer with your own family. You've achieved so much at such a young age— and now, to throw it all away for some foolish sentiment. It's a great pity."

Kuang Shi bit his lip to hold back his words, but he could not. "Serving my country's not a foolish sentiment. It is the highest duty!"

Lawrence Chung spoke up. "When did you become such a big-time patriot? Yesterday you were bragging about a six-figure income, and today you're Mr. Public Servant filled with humility. Who are you trying to kid, Charlie?"

Mrs. Yang was also unimpressed. "You want to be an idealist like your father? When we all chose to leave, he stayed behind. And look at him now." Carolyn tried to dissuade her mother but it was futile. "No! It's better he hears! I don't want a sentimental fool for a son-in-law!"

"Po Ling, you should not say that," Shiao Lin admonished her friend.

"What shouldn't I say? That I don't want my daughter to be imprisoned in China? That I don't want a son-in-law who spoils my dead husband's wealth?! What shouldn't I say?! Anyone who'd turn his back on one hundred thousand dollars a year is certainly a fool. And for what? For some stupid nationalism. What good has it done his father and mother living their last days in poverty?" Kuang Shi's heart burned.

"Please! Don't insult my parents!"

"Come. Carolyn, let's go before I insult everyone else." They gathered their belongings quickly and left without another word.

Shiao Lin wept bitterly. Everyone sat still, the silence only magnifying her loud sobs.

"Damn!" Lawrence Chung slammed his fist hard against his palm. He got up and moved over to the small sofa that had just been vacated. He looked at his wife, too angry to console her. "I told you not to arrange this meeting. But you wouldn't listen." His words only made Shiao Lin more grief-stricken. Susan brought her mother a handkerchief.

When she had composed herself, Shiao Lin turned to her nephew. "Do you know why I was pushing for this. Because..." Before she could finish she was again sobbing. Kuang Shi felt horrible. The last thing he wanted was to cause his aunt pain. He had to admit that he hadn't prepared them about his going to China. Did they really want him to marry Carolyn that badly?

Shiao Lin blurted out. "It's just that I don't want you to become a Hare Krishna monk."

"What?" Kuang Shi was mystified.

"Friday night your uncle and I were walking near Rockefeller Center, and there you were with all those crazy people! Those monks in their robes! Do you think I want you to be like that? Is there any mother in the world that would wish such a thing for her son?"

Lawrence Chung looked at his nephew. It was one thing to be naive about politicians, but quite another to be duped by religious sentiment. If his nephew couldn't hear what he had said earlier, he'd make certain that he'd understand him clearly now.

"How did you get mixed up with that group?"

Kuang Shi was already exhausted from the emotional strain of the past hour. Now he realized that he was heading for another tense session.

"I only met them a few weeks ago. I've read some of their books and attended one or two meetings." He wished his uncle would just drop the subject.

"You're a scientist. How can you believe in such stuff?"

"Their philosophy is logical. In fact, I'd say it's scientific."

"Jumping up and down in the street, screaming your head off is scientific? Is that what they gave you a Ph.D. for? What's gone wrong with you? Are you sick, or has something else happened to you we don't know about? I mean ... ," he paused to collect his thoughts. "Look, Charlie, let me tell you about these people. They're just beggars. They don't know what an honest day's work is. They just live off other people like leeches. It's the same with all religions. They speak some fancy philosophy to play with your mind, and before you know it they've got your intelligence, your money, and then your life."

Kuang Shi was too exhausted to protest. He just sat slumped on the sofa listening to his uncle go on.

"Okay, if you want to believe in God, that's fine. Nothing wrong with it. Some of the best people I know believe in God. Jimmy Allen is a Christian, and Arnold Rosen, you know the fellow who owns the jewelry shop next to the restaurant? He's a Jew. And most of the Chinese are either Buddhists or believe in Confucius or in something like that. I always say there's nothing wrong with religion if it makes you feel good." He leaned forward, his elbows on his knees. "But what I'm trying to say is, just don't take it too seriously. If you want to go to church or some temple once a week—fine. If you want to say a prayer every night—fine. But just don't let it carry you away so that it's all you think about day and night."

Kuang Shi sought to reassure his uncle and aunt. "Today I agreed to get married. Of course, I never expected everyone to react so strongly. At least you should be relieved that I was not thinking to become a monk."

"But the Hare Krishnas are all monks. They just beg for a living." Kuang Shi was not sure what to reply. He had only spoken about the philosophy with Sanatan Swami. He had never thought to ask such practical questions. But he doubted his uncle's version.

"I don't know," he said. "But I'll be careful, just as you've advised."

Shiao Lin got up and moved into the kitchen. She had prepared a big dinner, expecting to celebrate. It had turned out to be a day she wished she could forget.

Johnny turned on the TV, to a basketball game, Uncle Lawrence went upstairs, and Susan joined her mother in the kitchen. Kuang Shi sat thoughtfully, wondering what the reaction would be to his next announcement.

15

KUANG SHI SAT FORLORNLY, elbows pressed upon his desk, his head heavy with worry, resting on his fists. Adding to his already depressed spirits, the rain beat on the window panes. He thought of the saying, "April showers bring May flowers," but it didn't make him optimistic about the future. Things had to brighten, just as the rain would eventually stop, but when? And how?

He was too morose to want to see anyone. When Winston phoned, he excused himself on the plea of a headache. There was a note from Ann saying she wanted to see him, probably something in regard to David. But what help could he give?

He laughed half-heartedly, wishing he could do what he wanted, without caring what anyone else thought. But his life was not only his; there were others who had a share in it, and their needs and desires could not be denied.

Yet there was a broader issue involved, one that transcended family lines. He was a citizen of China, and the country seemed to want a share in his future. Absorbed in his studies these past five years in America, he didn't realize the depth of his attachment to his homeland. Assured of his Ph.D. degree, he had begun to relax for the first time in years and found himself deeply introspective.

Amidst the pressures of family, nation, and career, another force had begun to stir in his conscience. The galvanizing force of Krishna consciousness had increased his awareness of his spiritual needs. In a way, he considered it the catalyst of recent events. Indeed, it threatened to overpower all the others.

He picked up the *Bhagavad-gītā*, which he had been studying carefully. Lord Krishna, the Supreme Personality of Godhead, had assumed the position of a teacher in order to help His dear friend and devotee Arjuna. Kuang Shi realized that it was easy to identify with Arjuna's plight. He too was torn between his duties to family, nation, and God. Arjuna was a great soldier, but these conflicts within him stymied his ability to fight, and Krishna took this opportunity to teach the *Bhagavad-gītā*. Krishna chastised His student and called him a fool. Kuang Shi reflected for a moment; he himself was no less a fool. He was also bewildered, unable to determine the best course of action. Krishna quickly pointed to the source of Arjuna's confusion: he had mistaken the body to be the self and those related to the body to be his real self-interests, whereas it was the soul that was real, and the soul's service to God one's real self-interest. It struck Kuang Shi how true it was that happiness and distress, as well as fame and infamy, were as temporary as the coming and going of winter and summer seasons. He wondered if he could ever be as tolerant and undisturbed as Krishna told Arjuna to be. He, like Arjuna, found himself considering the consequence of his actions and their effect upon himself and those whom he loved, but it was impossible to satisfy everyone. That's why Arjuna had to act according to his duty, without attachment to the results.

It was a situation analogous to Kuang Shi's, for he, too, wanted to please his family and yet fulfill his duties. But how could he neglect either of them? Just as Arjuna had to fight and not run from the battlefield, so Kuang Shi realized that he too would have to act decisively—but if it came to deciding between his nation and his family, how could he choose? It was hard to properly understand the *Bhagavad-gītā*'s instructions. Yet, there was no reason to lament and therefore no reason to blame himself for his aunt's and uncle's grief. He tried to remember Krishna's instructions on the subject, and suddenly it occurred to him. No one caused another's suffering or enjoyment, for those were the results of each individual's present and past actions. At last, he was beginning to feel some relief. The *Bhagavad-gītā* was assuring him that his own life was not meant simply to fulfill the mundane needs and desires of others. Suddenly it dawned upon him that what was true for his family was equally true for his nation which was no more than an expanded family. And if it was true for them, it was just as true for humanity at large.

Had he been born to another family or another nation, Kuang Shi mused, the demands on him would have been entirely different—yet he would have been no more responsible for them than he was for the present ones. This principle was applicable under all circumstances, and that was the point. His birth had been determined by the actions and desires of his previous life. But all these desires— his, the family's, the nation's—were the result of ignorance, ignorance of spiritual identity. Remove the ignorance, erase material desires— this is what Krishna was telling Arjuna.

Kuang Shi recalled how bewildered he had been sitting amongst his relatives the previous day, his mind tossed about like a boat on turbulent waters. Arjuna had also complained to Krishna that it was impossible to control the mind by ordinary means. But Krishna informed His student that the mind could be made the best of friends rather than the worst of enemies if one controlled it by concentrating on Him.

Remembering the difficulties Arjuna had to face, Kuang Shi was trying to see his problems as insignificant. Krishna had advised Arjuna to practice mental control in the midst of a raging battle. But while Arjuna had succeeded, Kuang Shi had to admit that he had failed, despite the tiny battle that he had fought. Still, the war was not yet lost.

Taking the chanting beads in hand, Kuang Shi pushed

aside the desk chair and sat on the floor. His legs crossed and eyes closed, he began to chant: Hare Krishna, Hare Krishna, Krishna Krishna, Hare Hare / Hare Rama, Hare Rama, Rama Rama, Hare Hare. Over and over he repeated: Hare Krishna, Hare Krishna, Krishna Krishna, Hare Hare / Hare Rama, Hare Rama, Rama Rama, Hare Hare. Gradually his mind became absorbed in the transcendental sound vibration of the *mantra*. dissolving his melancholy entirely and driving away his anxieties. His heart lightened, his mind became pacified, soothed by Krishna's holy names.

16

KUANG SHI AND ANANTA continued to chant on their beads as they waited for Sanatan Swami. Though there were chairs in the room, Ananta sat on the floor and Kuang Shi followed his example. When the door opened and Sanatan Swami entered, Ananta offered his obeisances, and humbly Kuang Shi did the same.

"Oh, you're making advancement. Very good." Sanatan Swami was visibly pleased with Kuang Shi's behavior. He sat in one of the seats and smiled very pleasantly.

The composed presence of Sanatan Swami made Kuang Shi realize the degree of anxiety he had felt the past few days. Now he felt secure in the association of the spiritual master. Sanatan Swami was a study in serenity, the effect of full surrender to Krishna. He immediately inquired about Kuang Shi's well-being as well as that of his friends. He seemed to listen with great interest to their experiences of the past week. As Kuang Shi talked, Sanatan Swami occasionally inquired about specific details, hearing everything patiently and attentively.

Before Kuang Shi could articulate the question which

he had come to ask, Sanatan Swami spoke. "Human society is sometimes compared to a beehive, which is very appropriate because when bees try to enjoy the honey comb, they are bitten by other bees. Thus, their enjoyment of the honey is mixed with suffering.

"As bees collect pollen from various flowers, so humans try to secure money from various sources. And just as bees construct a hive, humans build individual homes, communities, cities, and nations. However, after these empires are created, these same builders are harassed by the bites of others. Within the home a man is bitten by all of his relatives' demands. In fact, one's relatives are sometimes compared to thieves, because a person earns his livelihood with great endeavor only to have it plundered by the rest of his family. Empires are created for the common enjoyment of all the citizens, yet as soon as they are built other nations become envious. Sometimes they declare war on one another, making such human beehives sources of great misery." Sanatan Swami began to laugh, and his two young students laughed with him.

"Although they're creating their beehives to enjoy the sweetness of their senses, at the same time they must suffer from the stings of others."

"What makes men so blind that they learn nothing from their past experiences?" Kuang Shi inquired.

"There are two classes of men: devotees and nondevotees. Nondevotees have acted sinfully in previous lives, and in this life their sinful actions continue. In the *Bhagavad-gītā* Krishna categorizes them thus:

> Those miscreants who are grossly foolish, who are lowest among mankind, whose knowledge is stolen by illusion, and who partake of the atheistic nature of demons do not surrender unto Me.

"Is there any hope for them?" Kuang Shi asked, thinking compassionately of his relatives. "Only if they are favored by a devotee."

"I don't understand."

Sanatan Swami was expert in studying the minds of others. Knowing that Kuang Shi was speaking of his own family, he spoke directly to him. "If you want to help those dear to you, then teach by your example. Don't try to discourage them in their present activities. Rather, as they are acting with attachment to results, you should perform your service in devotion, free of all attachment. By seeing your example they may gradually come to the proper realization, otherwise if you try to instruct them now they'll only become angry. When a snake is fed, it only increases its venom." It was difficult for Kuang Shi to hear his relatives compared to snakes but he had to admit that if he tried to instruct them they would certainly become angry. The recent meeting with them left no doubt about this in his mind.

Sanatan Swami was not satisfied that his young student had understood the point fully. He wanted to impress upon him the danger of mundane family attachments. "Family life is sometimes compared to being chained in prison. A man is chained to the charming beauty of a woman, by her solitary embraces and talks, and by the sweet words of his children. Thus illusioned, he forgets his eternal identity."

"Does one have to become a monk to make spiritual advancement?" Kuang Shi remembered the warning of his uncle.

Sanatan Swami was amused. "What do you think a monk is?" he asked.

"Someone who doesn't marry and instead of working, begs to earn his living."

"That's a stereotyped idea," began the master. "A better term for 'monk' is 'renunciant.' It does not depend on whether or not one is married. Renunciation refers to being unattached to the results of one's work while still performing it. We discourage laziness. Everyone must peacefully engage in service to the Supreme Lord.

"The public often thinks that renunciation is synonymous with begging. Perhaps in some cases that's true, but our Krishna conscious devotees don't beg. Instead, we give people books in exchange for their donations. In an advanced civilization renunciants and teachers are the most highly appreciated citizens and are supported for their work. Unfortunately, at the present time those who practice spiritual life full-time are often mistrusted. In any case, all our members are very active. Ananta, why don't you introduce Kuang Shi to Nitai. Nitai is one of my godbrothers," the Swami explained. "He's a businessman, married with two children. By meeting him you'll have the opportunity to see how one can be practically engaged in Krishna's service. Perhaps you have some questions you'd like to ask me?"

Kuang Shi thoughtfully formulated his questions. "From my reading of the *Bhagavad-gītā* and hearing you speak today, the essential lesson is that I must act without attachment to the results. I guess my question comes down to this: How should I act? What is my duty to my family and to my nation? And, how can I avoid attachment to the results?"

Sanatan Swami closed his eyes. He appeared to contemplate deeply. Kuang Shi somehow felt that the spiritual master was even consulting with Krishna directly. For his part, Kuang Shi prepared himself to be as receptive as possible, hoping to derive the greatest benefit from the master's words.

After a few moments, Sanatan Swami spoke, "Your general situation is not very different from most others, but in your case there is a particular factor which makes it unique. I think that Krishna has a special purpose of His own to fulfill through you. Please try to understand what that is." Kuang Shi listened with the utmost attention.

"Krishna's plan began to take shape with your very birth. By naming you Kuang Shi, it was as if your father knew the Lord's desire. While other fathers would look to their sons with selfish interests, your father seemed to have instilled in you a deep concern for others' well-being. One day I should like very much to meet him." Kuang Shi could not hold back his tears hearing his father appreciated by a person whom he esteemed most highly. He prayed that one day they might in fact meet.

"Compassion and the desire to serve humanity are the greatest gifts your father and mother could have given you. You are also indebted to your uncle and aunt. Their kindness has made it possible for you to reside in America. You must repay these debts to your family.

"A man's actions should somehow satisfy all his benefactors, such as the many professors and others who have helped you along the way. Perhaps more than most you have so much to be thankful for. It is due to Krishna's special favor upon you. Although the Lord maintains all living entities, He is especially inclined to look after His devotees, just as a gentleman loves all children but has special love for his own." Kuang Shi was surprised to hear himself referred to as a devotee.

"Yes, you're a devotee of Krishna. Your desire to serve your countrymen with your scientific training is the magnanimous side of your devotional character. Even your willingness to get married on the request of your relatives, when personally you had little inclination, was due to your not wanting to cause others to suffer,

"Therefore, what I really think Krishna has in mind for you is that you return to China." Kuang Shi looked astonished. "Yes, accept Dr. Zhang's offer! It is all Krishna's arrangement. While your relatives are considering their own family interests, while you were pondering how to best utilize your scientific abilities, and while the Chinese government was contemplating how you could be of greatest service to its people, Krishna alone had the all-conclusive plan.

"Return to China. But when you return, don't go merely as your father's son or as a research chemist. Go as Lord Krishna's representative. In other words, don't just bring back scientific technology; return with the greatest knowledge of all—knowledge of the self. Your government wants you to help your people, so give them the greatest gift of all—eternal life full of bliss and knowledge. Tell everyone that human life is meant to revive one's loving relationship with Krishna and to go back to one's original home in the spiritual world. In this way you will do the greatest benefit not only to your family and nation, but to all the world. For in the future, they will look to China. Let them see a nation whose greatest wealth is its Krishna consciousness.

"You're qualified, and I'm sure the Chinese people are ready to help you. Go with the blessings of Krishna and become the glory of your family and your nation."

Kuang Shi was stunned. Sanatan Swami had just told him that Krishna had a hand in directing the course of his life. Nothing had happened by accident; it had all transpired under the ultimate supervision of the Supreme Controller. He had asked about his duty, and he had been shown the supreme duty. He had asked how he could best help others, and he had been told to be the giver of supreme help. Without discouraging him from fulfilling his worldly obligations, Sanatan Swami was teaching him that everything would be accomplished in the context of fulfilling his spiritual obligations. At this point, he had no idea how this was to be accomplished, but he had no doubt in the authority of Sanatan Swami's request. He was Krishna's representative, and as such, hearing from him was as good as hearing from Krishna Himself.

"Do you have any further questions?" Sanatan Swami asked. Yes, there were many, but Kuang Shi needed time to reflect. The next step would be a big one.

17

ON THE WAY TO THEIR meeting with Nitai, Ananta described to Kuang Shi and Red Simon the success that Sanatan Swami's godbrother had had in applying the principles of Krishna consciousness philosophy to business enterprises. In only ten years' time he had established a number of small-scale industries, developed a computer sales network, marketed a natural food line, and opened three vegetarian restaurants.

When Ananta, Kuang Shi, and Red Simon met Nitai, he was in his office talking on the phone. Ananta immediately bowed down, showing him the respect due a godbrother of his spiritual master. Ananta introduced his friends and thanked Nitai for making time in his busy schedule. He explained why Sanatan Swami asked him to bring the others.

"There are many ways to serve Krishna," Nitai began. "Not everyone can be a full-time teacher. Sometimes, circumstances make that impossible. Nevertheless, one may have a strong desire to serve the Lord in other ways."

"If a person works for Krishna, is that just as good as teaching?" Red asked. Kuang Shi had been thinking the same question, especially after being requested by Sanatan Swami to dedicate himself to propagating Krishna consciousness to the people of his nation. He had put so much into becoming a scientist, and if his knowledge could be used in serving Krishna, that would be ideal. He listened carefully to Nitai's answer.

"Those who teach this philosophy to others are certainly dear to Krishna, since they've taken directly to the service of rescuing the conditioned souls and helping them to go back to the spiritual world. However, in the *Bhagavad-gītā* Krishna clearly states that anyone can attain perfection if they offer Him the results of their prescribed duties."

"Who prescribes these duties?" Kuang Shi asked.

Nitai was enthusiastic to speak the philosophy. He mentally thanked his godbrother, Sanatan Swami, for giving him this opportunity; these were intelligent young men, and he would do his best to help them understand the practical applications of Krishna consciousness. Nitai responded to Kuang Shi's question.

"Each person's duties are determined by his or her own innate abilities. It's really quite natural. Some are inclined to intellectual pursuits, others to administration, still others to mercantile endeavors. And finally there are laborers."

"But each person is equally respected if he uses his talents for serving Krishna, right?"

Nitai smiled at Kuang Shi, confirming his point with a nod of his head. "These divisions of labor are sometimes compared to the different parts of the body. For example, intellectuals are like the head of the body, administrators its arms, merchants and farmers its belly, and workers its legs. All the parts are important and interdependent."

Red was alert and clever. "But the head is the most important. If I had to sacrifice any part of my body, I wouldn't want to lose my head."

A doubt entered Kuang Shi's mind. "Hearing you describe the divisions of labor reminds me of Confucius' teachings in which society was rigidly stratified and where intellectuals and administrators were given preference. Most of the population, especially those who were laborers and farmers, suffered terribly, and from what I remember of my studies the same unfair system was also current in India."

"Every society throughout the world and throughout history always has these divisions, but the corruption of this system occurs when natural divisions of work are determined by birthright instead of by one's actual abilities. This happened in China as well as India—in fact, even in medieval Europe. The systems became so wicked and corrupt that revolutions occurred everywhere."

Kuang Shi wanted to make certain he understood. "So you do or don't uphold that system? I'm not clear. The *Gītā* prescribes it, doesn't it?"

"Yes, but it's not based on birth. If one's father happens to be a district court judge, does that automatically make one a judge as well? Of course not. One has to qualify oneself on one's own merit. Everyone has equal opportunity."

Kuang Shi was satisfied with his explanation.

"You must be making a pretty good profit," Red said, looking around at the handsome office.

"Whatever profit we make, fifty percent is donated to Krishna's service."

"Fifty percent!" Red was astonished. "How's that possible? How can you keep your business going if you give that much of the profit away?"

"That's a scriptural injunction which I've always followed. It's the secret of all our success. Krishna's making us successful because we are offering Him the results of our work. If we didn't serve Krishna by giving Him the results, the work would be karmic."

"I don't quite understand," Red said.

"When a person works for his own personal benefit, he becomes entangled in the complexities of material actions and reactions, or *karma*. When that same work is performed to please Krishna, the Lord neutralizes the material reactions and thus purifies the activity of its karmic nature."

"They never taught us that in business school," said Red, grasping it.

"That's a real shame. Simply teaching students to be expert businessmen, expert administrators, expert teachers, expert laborers is not a full education. But if everyone is taught to cooperate together for pleasing Krishna, then society becomes peaceful, prosperous, and ultimately liberated."

"You must be my *guru*," joked Red, "because you're talking my language."

Nitai chuckled and went on with his explanation of how to work for Krishna.

"Everyone advances in devotional service to Krishna at his own pace. In the twelfth chapter of the *Bhagavad-gītā*, Krishna nicely accommodates the different degrees of realization and surrender. See if you can figure out where you fit in.

> Just fix your mind upon Me, the Supreme Personality of Godhead, and engage all your intelligence in Me. Thus you will live in Me always, without a doubt.
>
> My dear Arjuna, O winner of wealth, if you cannot fix your mind upon Me without deviation, then follow the regulative principles of *bhakti-yoga*. In this way develop a desire to attain Me.
>
> If you cannot practice the regulations of *bhakti-yoga*, then just try to work for Me, because by working for Me you will come to the perfect stage.
>
> If, however, you are unable to work in this consciousness of Me, then try to act giving up all results of your work and try to be self-situated.

"In other words, at least one should be sympathetic to the propagation of Krishna consciousness. Devotees require financial help, so if one has sufficient money he can help by building an office or a center for teaching Krishna consciousness. He can contribute to the publication of Krishna conscious literature, and voluntary service like this will help him to come eventually to the standard, whereupon he will be able to follow more exactly other practices."

"That sounds right for me," Red admitted.

"The Vedic literatures are very broad in their vision of uplifting all the conditioned souls. Their advice is not exclusive, applicable to only a few. We often meet persons who find it difficult to engage directly in Krishna's service. Perhaps there are objections from their family, some social obligations, or some other impediments. But even these persons can still make spiritual advancement if they will give the results of their work to some good cause."

"Any cause?" Kuang Shi asked with some surprise.

"Yes. For example, if one were to help in the construction of a hospital or some other community service, this would be considered a good cause. Social service, community service, national service—so long one gives up the hard-earned results of his actions, his mind will gradually become purified. Then he will be able to understand Krishna consciousness."

This was indeed a broad-minded policy, Kuang Shi thought. His fellow countrymen could easily be encouraged in this way. In fact, most Chinese were already in the spirit of voluntarily dedicating themselves to the service of their nation.

"In China," he said, "people believe that sacrifice for their nation is the highest cause. Because of the great needs of our country, many have been doing this their whole lifetime."

"Then they're excellent candidates for Krishna consciousness," Nitai said, confirming what Kuang Shi had suspected. Kuang Shi was slowly realizing why Sanatan Swami was so convinced about China's spiritual future.

"As a businessman, what is your greatest challenge," asked Red. Nitai did not hesitate in his reply, "To remember Krishna under all circumstances is the real challenge."

"How do you do it?"

With that question Nitai became thoughtful. Finally he replied, "With the help of my family." It was not the answer Red expected. "In fact, I think it would be nice if you met my family. Are you free tomorrow evening?" Red said that he was going out of town for the rest of the week, but Kuang Shi was not only free, he was eager to come. Until now he had really associated only with members of the renounced order of life like Sanatan Swami and Ananta. This would be his first opportunity to mix intimately with a Krishna conscious family. Suddenly, he had an inspiration: Why not introduce David and Ann to Nitai? Seeing a Krishna conscious family might help them resolve their differences.

"I'm free tomorrow evening."

"Fine. Can you come around 7:00 p.m.?"

"Certainly. Would it be possible for me to bring two of my friends?"

"Of course. You're most welcome. Ananta, you'll come also?" Ananta was not one to pass up an invitation for dinner at Nitai's home. Nitai's wife, Padma, was famous for her excellent cooking.

"You're missing a great opportunity, Red," Ananta added, "Padma is an exceptional cook."

"Well, we'll have to make it up for him right now," Nitai said, reaching into his desk drawer and pulling out two vegetable-filled *samosas*.

18

KUANG SHI OWED CARLOS a visit. It wasn't so much that they were close friends, because Carlos didn't have too many friends. His angry nature kept people at a distance, and now his anger had landed him in the hospital.

"Those crazy kids. I tried to help them, and this is the thanks they gave me." Carlos lay in a hospital bed in a private room paid for by his parents, his head and chest heavily bandaged. He had been the victim of a brutal attack, the work of a crazed drug addict.

"Look what this idiotic government is doing to people," he continued. "These Americans think they own the world. They won't leave my country alone, and they don't leave the poor people in this country alone either. Freedom!" Carlos snorted. "It's a joke! There's no equality here. Justice for the rich and let the poor kill themselves off."

Kuang Shi sat silently. Carlos was raving even more than usual. Some of his statements were incoherent, which Kuang Shi attributed to the blow on his head. His verbal attacks were aimed at any and all authorities.

Kuang Shi wondered what good he could accomplish by his visit. He had come out of duty, to offer consolation. But what was the use? As he saw it, Carlos had always espoused violence, and now he'd gotten a taste of it himself. Kuang Shi reflected momentarily about the intricacies of the law of *karma*. Finally he decided to interrupt.

"Carlos, listen! Stop fighting! Can't you see what it's done to you? You're always so angry, but how has your anger helped you? How is it ever going to help anyone? In China they're no longer hateful. The so-called Cultural Revolution was a failure, and everyone regrets it. Hatred creates more problems than it solves. You've always asked me about China, but the China you worship no longer exists. The Chinese leaders are changing the country through peaceful reform, not through violence."

Carlos was sullen, his lips pressed tightly together. He was listening, but not agreeing. Kuang Shi wanted to speak about Krishna consciousness. It was his duty, even if Carlos didn't want to hear it.

"I've also wanted to help people. My whole life I thought like that, that the best I could do to help mankind was to find a cure to killer diseases like AIDS. Carlos, listen to me!" Kuang Shi's voice was emphatic, trying to break down his resistance. "I've realized that there is a greater disease than AIDS. It's infected everyone, all of us."

"What?" Carlos was puzzled.

"Ignorance. Yes, ignorance is the number one disease of the world. The whole human population has lost sight of its goal." As Carlos comprehended what Kuang Shi was intimating, he turned his head to the side, becoming distant. He had least expected to hear such ideas from his friend Charles. Charles was a scientist; the Chinese were leaders of the communist movement. What was Charles doing, teaching religion to him?

Kuang Shi was fed up. In a tone that surprised even himself, he let loose on the pitiful figure of the bandaged Carlos.

"Okay, Mr. Know-It-All, if you're so smart, why are you lying there half-dead? If you want solid proof of ignorance, just look at yourself in the mirror! How can you help anyone else if you can't even help yourself? You lie there with all your big talk about revolution..."

"Charles, stop! I'm not interested in your religion, or any other. The world has had enough religion. Marx was right calling it an opiate."

"You're following blindly, Carlos."

"We each have our own way, Charles. Go away, I'm

tired." Kuang Shi could see there was no use. He had tried. "Hare Krishna," he said and left.

19

DAVID'S ATTACHMENT TO ANN made it difficult for him to maintain his anger. They were again speaking, but there was an undeniable strain in the relationship. Had Ann been more flexible by nature, as David wished, she might have modified her resolve somewhat to practice Krishna consciousness strictly. But upon his return from Connecticut, he found her determined to pursue spiritual life. His brief study of the *Bhagavad-Gītā* had at least convinced him that the philosophy was sound, but he doubted its practicality.

However, David's views were being quickly modified in the association of Nitai and his family. Nitai's wife, Padma, was not only an excellent cook but a charming hostess as well. She was a strongly built woman, black-haired, dark-eyed, with high cheek bones that gave her an almost Oriental appearance, and she carried herself with a graceful loveliness. Her intelligence and vivacious personality were her great assets, making her very pleasant company. She was a fit match for her husband in all respects. Nitai and Padma had been married for eighteen years, and she had borne him two sons—Manu, fifteen, and Narayan, who was eleven.

Throughout the multicourse dinner, Padma had been entertaining the guests with some of the more adventurous of the family's experiences. The way in which they had sacrificed personal conveniences for a higher cause of Krishna consciousness reminded Kuang Shi of the hardships faced by early American pioneers and the folk heroes of China, who were distinguished for their sacrifice to serve their country.

Ann was imagining herself in such pioneering situations. Krishna consciousness offered exciting possibilities. As amused as he was by the narrations, David could never envision himself in such circumstances. Born to wealth, he preferred to view such struggles from a distance. They would make for an exciting novel or a movie, not for a peaceful life. That's what he wanted—a normal American household without too many surprises. There was only one hitch: Ann. Expecting to enjoy conventional American home life with Ann was like dreaming of tranquility while being tied to a box of dynamite. She was a high-strung thoroughbred, not a docile mare to be hitched to a village cart. Cupid must certainly have had a sense of humor to have made a match like theirs. Nitai and Padma seemed so compatible, whereas he and Ann were as opposite as two people could be. Still, "opposites attract" was a proven formula. Anyway, he wasn't about to give her up for anything.

At the moment, Ann was giving him a look as if to say, "Isn't Krishna conscious married life wonderful?" After dinner they moved into the living room and David thought that this might be the ideal occasion to ask some hard questions.

"What's the Krishna conscious view on sex?" David asked. Ann felt embarrassed by David's bluntness, but Kuang Shi understood that it was the only way for David to get free of his doubts.

Nitai and his wife were not at all offended. They had been asked such questions hundreds of times. Nitai explained, "Sex life in marriage should be regulated by religious principles and specifically for the purpose of propagating children."

"That's all? I mean, what about love? It's one of the most basic of human instincts."

"Do you think only humans enjoy sex? It's the most basic instinct for all living beings."

"Then what's wrong with it?"

"Did I say anything was wrong with it? Sex is proper if it's used for Krishna."

David was amused. Sex for Krishna?

Nitai elaborated, "Humans and animals are essentially the same except for one major difference: greater intelligence. Humans understand what they're doing, but animals act instinctively. When an animal sees a member of the opposite sex, it doesn't consider, 'Is this my mother? Is this my daughter?' There are no restrictions for animals, but humans are meant to discriminate. To begin with, there are responsibilities. Sex life within marriage is permissible, not otherwise."

"That's reasonable. I wouldn't argue with that," said David.

"The primary responsibility," Nitai added soberly, "is to realize that sex will probably produce a child."

"Unless one uses some contraceptive method."

"That's not normal."

"So, you're against birth control?" The question was Kuang Shi's. He was thinking of China's huge population.

"Our philosophy is 'birth control by self-control,' not by artificial means."

David couldn't see the point. "But what's wrong with the contraceptive method if it allows one to enjoy sex without pregnancy?"

"The married couple is meant to strive for liberation, not simply to increase their lusty activities and thus prolong their material existence."

"But these are natural desires, so how can one ever give them up?" David was perplexed.

"It is said that lust can never be satisfied by any amount of sense enjoyment, just as fire is never extinguished by a constant supply of fuel. A lusty person never loses his appetite for sex, no matter how many times he enjoys it. Such lusty materialists are compared to goats, because when goats are brought to slaughter they continue to have sex up to the very moment of death."

"That's a bit of an exaggeration to compare people to goats."

"No, actually it's not. A famous king of India, Akbar, once asked his minister how long it takes one to become free from the sex urge. The intelligent minister told him to follow quickly, along with his beautiful young daughter. He took them to a dying man, and when the king and the princess entered his room, the dying man ignored the king completely and gazed lustily at the princess."

"Alright," David conceded. "Then tell me, how do you manage to have sex life only when you want a child?"

Nitai turned to his wife, Padma, and asked her to answer.

"Husband and wife express their love by helping each other advance in spiritual life. They don't see each other as mere objects of sense gratification. Rather, they view each other as Krishna's servants, and one service they can offer Krishna is to conceive a Krishna conscious child."

"Could you explain what you mean by that," Ann requested. She understood but was asking on David's behalf.

Padma eagerly shared what she knew. "Consciousness is eternal and doesn't die with the death of the body. When the soul leaves the body at the time of death, it takes its next birth according to its consciousness. It's Krishna who arranges for the soul to be born to a father and mother of similar consciousness. Technically speaking, the soul first enters the sperm of the man and is impregnated into the womb of the woman, and thus the body is gradually developed around the soul. The point to realize is that it's not an accident that determines which child is born to which parents. They are matched by consciousness.

"Understanding this science, Krishna conscious parents make every effort to purify their consciousness before attempting to conceive a child, and the result is that their children are very special. Parents of advanced consciousness have children of similarly advanced consciousness. That's the formula."

She studied David to make certain he was understanding. "When children are born from lusty desire only—in other words when they are born to parents who are simply enjoying sex for pleasure, they are described as *varna-sankara*, burdens to society. Children of this sort are heavily influenced by ignorance and passion, just as their parents were at the time of having sex."

David had been listening carefully. He was beginning to realize that there was a Krishna conscious answer to all questions. He was also beginning to realize that everything the devotees did was based on a thorough-going philosophy which included all aspects of life.

"How do a husband and wife help each other to stay Krishna conscious?" he asked, this time more submissively.

Padma continued to speak, "We rise early in the morning. Because we live far from any Krishna conscious center, we perform our spiritual discipline at home. After showering and dressing in clean clothes, we chant the Hare Krishna *mantra* to music. Then we chant sixteen rounds of the *mantra* on our beads. Next we read together from the *Bhagavad-gītā* or other devotional literatures. Finally, we end the program by eating sanctified food that we have offered to Krishna."

"How long does it take?" Ann asked.

"About three hours," said Padma. "It keeps us Krishna conscious throughout the day."

"How long did it take you to become such a good cook," David asked, changing the subject.

"No longer than it will take Ann," said Padma, smiling.

It was easy for Kuang Shi to see why Nitai had said his family was such a big help in his Krishna conscious career. His wife was as good a devotee as he and appeared to be an equally good teacher. He was also appreciating the importance of associating with advanced devotees like Nitai and Padma. Their experience and personal realizations made the *Bhagavad-gītā*'s teachings come to life. Kuang Shi had previously thought that Sanatan Swami was the only teacher of Krishna consciousness, but now he realized that there were many. Spreading Krishna consciousness was not one man's work. How many teachers were needed for the five billion humans on the planet, one quarter of them Chinese? Who was going to try to give them Krishna consciousness? The answer was clear. The only question was, how?

20

AS KUANG SHI MOUNTED the steps to Sanatan Swami's room, he felt as though he were leaving behind the world he knew and entering a new world, a new life. The feeling began last night when he and Winston, along with David and Ann, had arrived at the temple to stay for an entire weekend. Packing his bag, he had taken few personal effects. He thought to take an extra set of clothes, some books to study, but rejected these, at last settling on a toothbrush, a towel, and his *Bhagavad-gītā*. It was a symbolic act of renunciation, a willful desire to leave behind the things which reminded him of the past. The weekend at the temple was not to be merely a spiritual retreat; he felt as if he were about to take a new birth.

After his first night at the temple, he rose early in the morning and took a shower, but the bathing was more than a mere cleansing of his body, and as he joined the others in the temple for the early morning kirtan, he danced and chanted with a clean consciousness and an untainted heart. The experience made him feel as if he had removed the last vestiges of material attachment. As he ascended the stairs, he felt so free he thought he could fly.

He knocked on the door and heard the soft voice of Sanatan Swami beckoning. He opened the door slightly. The master was seated on a cushion, his effulgent saffron-robed form glowing in the soft lamp light. Kuang Shi silently closed the door, came forward, and prostrated himself in unconditional surrender.

When he sat up, he beheld the worshipable form of the spiritual master as never before. His vision was anointed with love and devotion for that person who had helped him remove the covering of ignorance from his heart. He listened to Sanatan Swami murmur the Hare Krishna *mantra*, only his fingers slightly moving on the wooden beads. Besides the chant, there was no other sound. Then Sanatan Swami spoke with a voice that filled the room.

"So, what is your decision?" There was no formal greeting, no other words. Just, "What have you decided?" What else was there to say?

With clarity of purpose and a voice laden with devotion, Kuang Shi said, "I want to offer myself to Krishna." It was an answer that said everything, the conclusion of weeks of searching, no doubt of lifetimes. There were no more qualms, no misgivings, just unconditional surrender.

"And what about your family?" Kuang Shi felt the teacher examining his determination. "I telephoned China."

"China?"

"Yes. I spoke with my father." There was silence except for the sound of the wooden beads moving between Sanatan Swami's fingers. "I told him of the offer of the Chinese government. My father is a great patriot and told me to accept the offer without question, even if some relatives were offended."

"Did you discuss Krishna consciousness at all?"

"No, I thought it would be best to wait until I go to China. I think my father will not only encourage me; he himself will take an interest in Krishna."

"And your uncle?"

"He was very disappointed. But what could he do when both my father and I were of the same opinion?"

Though Kuang Shi had no doubts, Sanatan Swami sought to reassure him further. "Your uncle and aunt may not realize it, but they will share in the benefits of your service to Krishna. It was they who helped you stay in America, and it was here that you got the opportunity to learn about Krishna. Krishna will reward them for the help they gave you now that you've become a devotee." Sanatan Swami chuckled to himself.

"What about the lady and her daughter you agreed to marry?"

"When she heard that I might be returning to China, she lost all interest in having me as a son-in-law."

Sanatan Swami began to smile and his smile kept increasing as if there was no end to his happiness. At last he said. "Lord Krishna has personally delivered you. You are not ordinary. You are the representative of a most important nation. Therefore Krishna has taken a personal hand in directing the course of your life. It is normally very difficult for a person to overcome his attachment to family, career, and nationality, yet you have very quickly transcended all of these. The only explanation is the causeless mercy of Krishna."

"I think it is your causeless mercy that has made it so easy," said Kuang Shi with heartfelt appreciation. "Because you desired that I become Krishna conscious, Krishna has made it very easy for me. I'm an ordinary person, a materialistic scientist, but you have transformed me from a Dr. Frog to a devotee of Krishna. How can I ever repay you?"

Within his mind Sanatan Swami repeatedly thanked Lord Krishna. He had prayed that the Lord accept this young man. With tears in his eyes he said, "Our meeting was arranged by providence. My spiritual master, Śrīla Prabhupāda, desired that Lord Chaitanya's prophecy be fulfilled. He often spoke about the Chinese people. He said that they would be the last to take to Krishna consciousness, but that once they took it up they would be the strongest devotees in the world. Lord Chaitanya predicted that the holy names of Krishna would be chanted in every town and village throughout the world. That prophecy was fulfilled except for the towns and cities of China. Now they too will be blessed. The prediction that the Chinese people would take to Krishna consciousness is not recent. The ancient *Vedas* clearly mention that the Chinese people will become purified of all sins by taking shelter of the devotees of the Lord:

> kirāta-hūṇāndhra-pulinda-pulkaśā
> ābhīra-śumbhā yavanāḥ khasādayaḥ
> ye 'nye ca pāpā yad-apāśrayāśrayāḥ
> śudhyanti tasmai prabhaviṣṇave namaḥ

Kirāta, Hūṇa, Andhra. Pulinda, Pulkaśa, Ābhīra, Śumbha, Yavana, members of the Khasa races and even others addicted to sinful acts can be purified by taking shelter of the devotees of the Lord, due to His being the supreme power. I beg to offer my respectful obeisances unto Him.

Sanatan Swami looked at Kuang Shi. "'Khasa' refers to the Chinese people. Now do you understand why my conviction about China is so strong? It is the prediction of the *Vedas*, the prediction of Lord Chaitanya, and the desire of my spiritual master. Their words can never fail."

Though Kuang Shi was feeling blissful, he still had many practical questions. "I have full faith in your instructions," he began, "so please help me to understand what part I may play to fulfill this prediction. There're many differences between China and America, basic freedoms and facilities which Americans take for granted but which may not be available to me in China. For example, I have my own room at Columbia University. But what if I have to share a room with someone else at Beijing?"

"It's best if you request the hospital to grant you your own room. After all, you're going to be the chief of research. But if they can't make such an arrangement, you can still practice Krishna consciousness, rising early at least four hours before you begin your work."

"I hope the staff's quarters have showers. As you noticed, some of the student quarters don't, and the bath houses are often open only during the daylight hours."

"It's essential that you shower after waking up in the morning. Somehow you have to find a way to do this. It's part of being Krishna conscious."

Kuang Shi was considering how he would chant if he had to share a room with someone else who was not Krishna conscious. "How will I chant Hare Krishna if my roommate is sleeping?"

"Chant softly. Or, when the weather is warm you can chant outdoors. The campus should be very peaceful at 5:00 a.m."

"Now I chant some of my rounds in the morning and some in the evening. Is it alright to maintain that schedule?"

"It's best to chant your rounds early in the morning. Once the day's activities begin it is difficult to concentrate on chanting. If possible, try to finish all your rounds before going to work. And after chanting, you should read. If you have rounds left over, you can chant them in the evening."

"What about my eating? The hospital certainly isn't going to provide me with vegetarian meals."

"Then you'll have to do your own cooking."

"But I don't know how to cook."

"Vegetarian cooking is easy to learn. Ananta can teach you. Sometimes when I travel I cook for myself in the hotel room. All it takes is a hotplate and a pot. It may be simple, but if you cook and offer it all to Krishna with devotion, it always turns out tasty and nourishing."

"What books should I read?" Kuang Shi asked.

Sanatan Swami considered for a moment and then replied, "The *Bhagavad-gītā* and the *Śrīmad-Bhāgavatam*. Śrīla Prabhupāda translated nearly one hundred books, so gradually you have to read all of them."

"Over the past few weeks I've realized how important it is to associate with devotees. Ann and David were not getting along, but by associating with Nitai and Padma they seemed to have worked out most of their problems. But I'll be all alone in China. Whom will I associate with?"

Sanatan Swami smiled. "You have to make some of the Chinese people Krishna conscious. Then the problem of association will be solved."

"But that may take some time," objected Kuang Shi.

"There are two types of association: vapu and vani. Vapu means 'physical association,' and vani means 'association through sound.' Of the two, physical association is not as important because it may not always be available. But association through sound, through hearing, is always available. The *Śrīmad-Bhāgavatam* describes the lives of the greatest devotees in history, and by reading it every day you can have the association of all of these great devotees. This is association through sound."

Kuang Shi was thoughtful. Based on what he had just heard from Sanatan Swami, he was confident he could maintain his own Krishna consciousness. But he was not so certain that he could induce others to accept the spiritual principles.

"How can I teach others about Krishna consciousness?" he asked. "In New York you have this cultural center where people can come and learn. And there are exhibitions like the Festival of India to attract the public. In fact, just your dress alone attracts attention. But I'll have to dress normally." Sanatan Swami appreciated Kuang Shi's practical question. He tried to give him reassurance.

"Your clothing is not very important. Dress according to your situation. You're a scientist and will be occupying an important position, so you have to dress appropriately. Now, as far as the books are concerned, they're the most important way to introduce your countrymen to the philosophy. One of the first services you can do after establishing your department is to get the government to approve our books."

"I don't think that will be very easy," said Kuang Shi.

"Why not?" Sanatan Swami responded immediately. "We're not teaching a sectarian dogma. These books are of reason, meant to benefit everyone. They are morally uplifting. The government should be happy if the citizens read our books. There is nothing political in them."

"But even if the government approves the books, who will pay for their printing? I wouldn't be able to sponsor the printing with the small salary I would be earning."

"I'm sure our Book Trust would be willing to sponsor the first printing. Once you have the books, you could sell them and use the profit to print more."

"So I should do everything legitimately, with government approval?"

"Did you know that the Soviet Union has recently given its official approval to Krishna consciousness? At first they arrested the Russian devotees, but later on, when they understood the philosophy and saw that it was extremely moral and beneficial, they gave their official approval. Now they have registered a Soviet Krishna consciousness society." Kuang Shi was amazed to hear this. During his student days in Beijing, some of his friends had taken part in protests, but he had always refused. He preferred to do everything in an authorized way.

"I think the Chinese government will at least be as reasonable as the Russians," continued Sana-tan Swami. "I think their main insistence will be that you register a society which is wholly Chinese and does not have any connection or affiliation to an international organization. That would be fine."

"But what if it takes some time for them to recognize the value of Krishna consciousness?" Kuang Shi tried to foresee all the difficulties he might face.

"A devotee must be patient but determined. He must pursue Krishna consciousness under all circumstances. There have been many instances when devotees were pressured to give up Krishna consciousness but refused. Try to persuade them with sound logic. Ultimately, you have to depend upon Krishna."

"How much attention should I give to my work?"

"You should give your full attention. Your government is depending on you to establish an important department of research. You shouldn't disappoint them in any way. If you can distinguish yourself in your field of activities, that in itself will be the best recommendation for Krishna consciousness."

Kuang Shi was satisfied with Sanatan Swami's practical instructions.

"Is there anything else?" Sanatan Swami asked.

"Yes, there is one more thing. Would you accept me as your disciple?" In his heart he had already accepted Sanatan Swami as his spiritual master. Now he wanted confirmation that Sanatan Swami was accepting him. If he was going to return to China, he wanted his final assurance.

Sanatan Swami gave his unhesitating reply. "I shall be happy to accept you on behalf of all the previous spiritual masters, and ultimately on behalf of the Supreme Lord Krishna. May you become fully Krishna conscious." Kuang Shi was speechless. Not knowing what else to do, he offered his obeisances.

"The sun is rising," said Sanatan Swami. "Draw open the curtains." Kuang Shi sprang up and ran to open the curtains. The golden rays of the morning sun brightened the room.

"Call all your friends here," Sanatan Swami ordered. Kuang Shi ran to the door with excitement. Before leaving he remembered to offer his obeisances again. Now he knew how Ananta felt when receiving the spiritual master's orders. It was the most wonderful and natural of feelings, an intrinsic quality of the soul.

Kuang Shi ran so quickly that he bumped full speed into Winston. Kuang Shi was astonished to see Winston wearing the saffron dress of a devotee. "Winston, what are you doing dressed in robes?" said Kuang Shi, as much surprised as appreciative. The combination of his black beard, the saffron robes, and his impressive size gave Winston an extraordinary appearance.

"You look like an ancient Chinese sage," Kuang Shi added.

Recovering after a moment's embarrassment, Winston explained. "They told me if I wanted to work in the kitchen, I had to wear one of these. I like it. What about you?" he said. "If you put on these robes, we'll actually have a Chinese sage here." Kuang Shi laughed.

"Think of what the public would say, Winston. A scientist in monk's robes? Philosophers like you can get away with anything, but we scientists are respectable people. Where are Ann and David?"

"Here we are," said Ann cheerfully as she turned the corner of the stairs, followed by David and Ananta. "How do you like my sari?" Ann was dressed in the traditional Vedic sari.

"Very elegant," Winston said with appreciation. "These clothes are so much more comfortable than Western dress."

"Devotional clothing is neither Eastern nor Western," corrected Ananta. "The same style of clothing is worn in the spiritual world."

"Sanatan Swami wants to see all of us," announced Kuang Shi. "He's waiting for us." Without delay they all ran up the stairs eagerly and burst into his room.

The majestic figure of Sanatan Swami stood before them, and as they sat in his presence they felt just like children, secure in the shelter of their loving father. He gazed at them, marveling at how each had been transformed by Krishna consciousness. He quoted from the *Bhagavad-gītā*:

> *bahūnāṁ janmanām ante*
> *jñānavān māṁ prapadyate*
> *vāsudevaḥ sarvarm iti*
> *sa mahātmā su-durlabhaḥ*

After many births and deaths, he who is actually in knowledge surrenders unto Me, knowing Me to be the cause of all causes and all that is. Such a great soul is very rare.

"From our first meeting I could understand that you were all intelligent and that with the proper encouragement you would be able to surrender to Krishna. If we always remember that Krishna is the cause of all causes, then we will see Krishna everywhere and in all circumstances. If one loves one's child and sees the child's clothes or playthings, he or she will immediately remember the child, 'Oh, these are my child's clothes. These are my child's playthings.' This is the nature of love. If one actually loves Krishna, one will remember Him always because everything belongs to Krishna. Krishna describes how He may be always remembered:

> All that you do, all that you eat, all that you offer and give away, as well as all austerities that you may perform, should be done as an offering unto Me.

"Such a person is fully Krishna conscious, and Krishna reciprocates by never forgetting the devotee. A pure devotee is just like a precious jewel kept in the hand of the Lord. When you hold something precious in your hand, you are very careful, and similarly Krishna holds the devotee and takes special care of him.

"Always try to engage in Krishna's service twenty-four hours a day through hearing, chanting, remembering, offering prayers, worshiping, serving His lotus feet, rendering others service, becoming His friend, or surrendering fully to Him. If you are sincere, Krishna will give you all the assistance you need. Even if you experience some difficulty or make some mistake, Krishna will overlook it and help you to rectify yourself. Be patient and learn to be temperate in all your habits of eating, sleeping, working, and recreation. In this way you will mitigate all your material pains and anxieties.

"Devotional service to Krishna is eternal. Whether one

performs it in this world or in the spiritual world, the activity is one and the same. Devotional service does not change, it only becomes sweeter. In the beginning a devotee renders devotional service under the guidance of the spiritual master, following the rules and regulations, but when the devotee becomes mature in realization, he renders service directly in association with the Supreme Lord. The service is the same, but it becomes sweeter and more relishable as one progresses in realization."

As Sanatan Swami concluded, each of them felt indebted. Winston expressed their feelings, "I think we all feel very grateful for the kindness you have shown us. We know how busy you are, yet you have gone out of your way to offer us Krishna consciousness."

"I've simply done my duty, but you should be grateful to your friend Kuang Shi. Due to him we have all had the opportunity to meet." Sanatan Swami looked at Kuang Shi. "Have you told them of your decision?" Seeing that he had not, Sanatan Swami urged him to speak.

Kuang Shi was uncertain how to begin. They had been his friends since he had first come to America. Once he returned to China, it was not certain whether he would ever see them again. "You have been my best friends for many years," he began, but faltered, unable to continue.

"Charles, what's wrong?" Ann asked. She could see that Kuang Shi was overcome with emotion.

Kuang Shi gained control of himself. "It's not easy to say this," and again he paused, "I'm returning to China."

"When are you coming back?" Winston's voice was anxious. Kuang Shi was unable to respond.

"Is there some problem, Charles?"

"No, there's nothing wrong, except that I feel bad to be leaving. About two weeks ago a representative of the Chinese government approached me and asked that I return to my country. They want me to establish an AIDS research department at one of the most important hospitals in China. I'm to be chief of research. In America I'm a small fish in a big pond. But in China there are very few with my qualifications."

"Well, that's just fine," said David in a way that made it clear that it wasn't fine at all. "After practically pushing us into Krishna consciousness, now you're deserting us."

Kuang Shi felt horrible. He looked to his spiritual master for help. Seeing Kuang Shi overcome with emotion, Sanatan Swami soothed their feelings.

"You shouldn't blame Kuang Shi, nor should you feel disappointed. One must do one's duty, even though it may not always please others."

"I don't understand," said Winston.

"The sense of duty is not very much understood in America today, but in China it is still very strongly felt by nearly everyone. You call Kuang Shi 'Charles' and perhaps you've never inquired what his real name means. 'Kuang' means 'wide' or 'plentiful,' and 'Shi' means 'to give in charity.' Kuang Shi means 'one who gives abundantly.' "

"That's a beautiful name," said Ann. "Why did you ever use 'Charles'?" Kuang Shi smiled, but before he could answer, Sanatan Swami spoke again.

"That's the very same question I asked when we first met. He had stopped using the name given to him by his father. His father is a very patriotic gentleman and wished that his son give his life for serving others, but not until he found out about Krishna consciousness did he really understand the full import of his name.

"Kuang Shi's return to China is not merely to fulfill worldly obligations. It's actually Krishna's desire. Krishna wants Kuang Shi to give Krishna consciousness to all his countrymen. The ancient *Vedas* specifically mention the Chinese among the races of the world who will take to Krishna consciousness. Lord Chaitanya also predicted that Krishna's glories would be chanted in every town and village, and Śrīla Prabhupāda, my spiritual master, requested us to fulfill Lord Chaitanya's prophecy. So Kuang Shi's return to China isn't due to selfish motivation. He will be fulfilling the words of previous spiritual masters and of Krishna Himself." There was a silence as they tried to comprehend the will of destiny. At last Ann spoke out.

"Well, I think it's great! You have my full support, Charl ... I mean Kuang Shi," Ann smiled, correcting herself.

There was a sudden knock on the door. Ananta opened the door, and to everyone's surprise. Red entered.

"So here you all are." he said. "You're having a party and you didn't even think to invite me. Real friends!"

"We thought you had gone out of town," Kuang Shi apologized.

"No excuses, no excuses," Red said, though it was clear he was not really offended. "I've brought something for you, Maharaj." Red walked straight to where Sanatan Swami was seated and handed him an envelope, and then, to everyone's surprise, he bowed and touched his head to the floor. Taking his seat among the others he requested Sanatan Swami to open the envelope.

Sanatan Swami opened it neatly at one end. Inside he found a check, a donation for ten thousand dollars. Sanatan Swami smiled broadly, reading the amount aloud to all of the assembled devotees.

"Wow!" said Winston.

"That's nothing," said Red. "There will be a lot more coming in the future. Maybe I can't be a devotee, but at least I can give whatever I can."

"Oh, you're very much a devotee," Sanatan Swami reassured him.

"Charles is leaving us," David said.

"Where are you going?" Red asked.

"China," David said.

"When?" Red wanted to know.

"I guess as soon as I receive my degree, probably in two months."

"Two months. Hmmm," Red was thoughtful. "What's it like in Beijing? I mean, what's the weather like in June or July?"

"About the same as it is in New York," Kuang Shi answered. "A bit warm, but still quite pleasant."

"And are there any modern hotels?" Everyone laughed. "Just like New York." Kuang Shi said.

"Okay," Red said decisively. "We're all going."

"What?" Winston wondered if he had heard him correctly.

"You heard me, I said we are all going. The party is on me. I'll pay for everything. How can we let our brother Charles return alone?"

"Red Simon, is this just another one of your jokes?" Ann asked, hoping it wasn't.

"My word is as good as gold," said Red. There was an outburst of joy. Everyone was talking at once.

"If this isn't the spiritual world, it's as close as I've ever been," said Winston.

"This is love," confirmed Sanatan Swami.

"And this is the real meaning of spiritual life," said Kuang Shi, as tears of happiness streamed from his eyes.

Hare Krishna Centers
In North America, Australia & New Zealand
2001

EUROPE
UNITED KINGDOM AND IRELAND
Belfast, Northern Ireland Brooklands, 140 Upper Dunmurray Lane, BT17 OHE/ Tel. +44 (01232) 620530
Birmingham, England 84 Stanmore Rd., Edgbaston, B16 9TB/ Tel. +44 (0121) 420-4999
Coventry, England Kingfield Rd., Radford, West Midlands (mail: 19 Gloucester St., CV1 3BZ)/ Tel. +44 (01203) 552822
Glasgow, Scotland Karuna Bhavan, Bankhouse Rd., Lesmahagow, Lanarkshire, ML11 0ES/ Tel. +44 (01555) 894790/ Fax: +44 (01555) 894526/
Liverpool, England 114A Bold St., Merseyside, L1 4HY/ Tel. +44 (0151) 512-9319
London, England (city) 9-10 Soho St., W1D 3DL/ Tel. +44 (020) 437-3662; residential /pujaris, 7439-3606; shop, 7287-0269;
London, England (country) Bhaktivedanta Manor, Dharam Marg, Hilfield Lane, Watford, Herts, WD2 8EZ/ Tel. +44 (01923) 857244/ Fax: +44 (01923) 852896
London, England (south) 42 Enmore Road, South Norwood, SE25/ Tel. +44 (0181) 656-4296 or 654-3138
Manchester, England 20 Mayfield Rd., Whalley Range, M16 8FT/ Tel. +44 (0161) 226-4416/ Tel. & fax: +44 (0161) 860-6117/
Northern Ireland Govindadvipa Dhama, ISKCON Inisrath Island, BT92 9GN, Co. Fermanagh/ Tel. +44 (013657) 21512 or

ADDITIONAL RESTAURANT
Dublin, Ireland Govindas Restaurant, 4 Aungier St., Dublin 2/ Tel. +353 (01) 475-0309
GERMANY
Abentheuer Boeckingstr. 8, 55767/ Tel. +49 (06782) 980436/ Fax: 980437
Cologne Taunusstr. 40, 51105/ Tel. +49 (0221) 830-1241/ Fax: +49 (0221) 837-0485
Heidelberg Forum 5, Wohnung 4, 69126/ Tel. +49 (06221) 384553
Munich Wachenheimer Strasse 1, 81539/ Tel. +49 (089) 6880-0288/ Fax: +49 (089) 6880-0289
Nuremberg Kopernikusplatz 12, 90459/ Tel. +49 (0911) 446-7773
RURAL COMMUNITY
Jandelsbrunn (Nava Jiyada Nrsimha Ksetra) Zielberg 20, 94118/ Tel +49 (08583) 316/ Fax: +49 (08583) 1671
ITALY
Asti Frazione Valle Reale 20, 14018 Roatto (AT)/ Tel. +39 (0141) 938406

Bergamo Villaggio Hare Krishna, 24040 Chignolo dIsola (BG)/ Tel. +39 (035) 494-0706/ Fax: +39 (035) 494-0705
Bologna Via Ramo Barchetta 2, Castagnolo Minore, 40010 Bentivogolio (BO)/ Tel. +39 (051) 863924
Milan Centro Culturale Govinda, Via Valpetrosa 5, 20123/ Tel. +39 (02) 862417
Rome Hare Krishna Forum, Piazza Campo de Fiori 27, 00186/ Tel. +39 (06) 683-2660
Vicenza Prabhupada-desa, Via Roma 9, 36020 Albettone (VI)/ Tel. +39 (0444) 790573/ Fax: +39 (0444) 790581

RURAL COMMUNITY
Florence (Villa Vrindavan) Via Comunale Scopeti 108, 50026 San Casciano in Val di Pesa (FI)/ Tel. +39 (055) 820054/ Fax: +39 (055) 828470

ADDITIONAL RESTAURANT
Milan Govindas, Via Valpetrosa 5, 20123/ Tel. +39 (02) 862417
SPAIN
Barcelona Plaza Reial 12, Entlo 2, 08002/ Tel. +34 (93) 302-5194
Madrid Espritu Santo 19, 28004/ Tel. +34 (91) 521-3096
Malaga Ctra. Alora, 3, Int., 29140 Churriana/ Tel. +34 (95) 262-1038

RURAL COMMUNITY
Guadalajara (New Vraja Mandala) (Santa Clara) Brihuega/ Tel. +34 949 280436
RESTAURANT
Barcelona Restaurante Govinda, Plaza de la Villa de Madrid 4-5, 08002/ Tel. +34 (93) 318-7729

SWEDEN
Gothenburg Tr_dgardsgŒtan 6, 41108/ Tel. +46 (031) 879648
Lund Bredgatan 28 ipg, 22221/ Tel. +46 (046) 399500/ Fax: +46 (046) 188804
Stockholm Fridhemsgatan 22, 11240/ Tel. +46 (08) 654-9002/ Fax: +46 (08) 650-8813
Stockholm (country) Radha-Krishna Temple, K_rsnŒs GŒrd, 14792 Gro_dinge, Tel. +46 (08) 53029800/ Fax: +46 (08) 53025062
Uppsala ISKCON, 74193 Knivsta/ Tel. +46 (018) 102924

RURAL COMMUNITY
J_rna Almviks Gard, 15395/ Tel. +46 (08) 55152050/ Fax: +46 (08) 55152060

RESTAURANTS

Stockholm Govindas, Fridhemsgatan 22, 11240/ Tel. +46 (08) 654-9002/ Fax: +46 (08) 650-8813
Lund Govindas, Bredgatan 28 ipg, 22221/ Tel. +46 (046) 120413/ Fax: +46 (046) 188804

SWITZERLAND

Basel St. Jakob-Strasse 33, 4132 Muttenz/ Tel. & fax: +41 (061) 462-0614
Lugano Via Borghese 12, 6600 Locarno/ Tel. +41 (091) 752-3851/ Fax: +41 (091) 751-3852
Zurich Bergstrasse 54, 8030/ Tel. +41 (01) 262-3388/ Fax: +41 (01) 262-3114

ADDITIONAL RESTAURANT

Zurich Govindas, Preyergasse 16, 8000/ Tel. +41 (01) 251-8859

OTHER COUNTRIES

Amsterdam, The Netherlands Van Hilligaertstraat 17, 1072 JX/ Tel. +31 (020) 675-1404/ Fax: +31 (020) 675-1405
Antwerp, Belgium Amerikalei 184, 2000/ Tel. +32 (03) 237-0037
Bucharest, Romania str. Laborator, No. 124, Bl. 40, Ap. 95/ Tel. +40 (1) 350-3575 or +40 (56) 191565
Copenhagen (Hiller¿d), Denmark Baunevej 23, 3400 Hiller¿d/ Tel. +45 4828-6446/ Fax: +45 4828-7331
Helsinki, Finland Ruoholahdenkatu 24 D (III krs) 00180/ Tel. +358 (9) 694-9879/ Fax: +358 (9) 694-9837
Iasi, Romania Stradela Moara De Vint 72, 6600
Kaunas, Lithuania 37, Savanoryu pr./ Tel. +370 (7) 22-2574 or 26-8953/ Fax: +370 (7) 70-6642
Kokosovce, Slovak Republic Abranovce 60, 08252 Kokosovce/ Tel. +421 (51) 7798482
Lisbon, Portugal Rua Dona Estefania, 91 R/C 1000 Lisboa/ Tel. & fax: +351(01) 314-0314 or 352-0038
Ljubljana, Slovenia Zibertova 27, 1000/ Tel. +386 (061) 131-2124/ Fax: +386 (061) 310815
Paris, France 31 rue du docteur Jean Vaquier, 93160 Noisy le Grand/ Tel. & fax: +33 (01) 4303-0951
Plovdiv, Bulgaria ul. Prosveta 56, Kv. Proslav, 4015/ Tel. +359 (032) 446962
Porto, Portugal Rua S. Miguel 19, 4050-560 (mail: Apartado 4108, 4002-00)/ Tel. & fax: (351) 222-007-223
Prague, Czech Republic Jilova 290, Praha 5 - Zlicin 155 21/ Tel. +42 (02) 5795-0391 or -0401/ Fax: +42 (02) 302-1628
Croatia, Croatia Vinkuran centar 58, 52000 (mail: P.O. Box 16)/ Tel. & fax: +385 (052) 573581
Radhadesh, Belgium Chateau de Petite Somme, 6940 Septon-Durbuy/ Tel. +32 (086) 322926/ Fax: +32 (086) 322929
Riga, Latvia 56, K. Baron st., LV1011/ Tel. +371 (02) 27-2490/ Fax: +371 (2) 27-4120
Rijeka, Croatia Sv. Jurja 32, 51000 (mail: P.O. Box 61)/ Tel. +385 (051) 543 055/ Fax: +385 (051) 543 056
Sarajevo, Bosnia-Herzegovina ISKCON, Gornjo Vakufska 12, 71000/ Tel. +387 (071) 201530
Skopje, Macedonia Vvz. ÒISKCON,Ó Roze Luksemburg 13, 91000/ Tel. +389 (091) 201451
Sofia, Bulgaria 4 ÒF.J.KjuriÓ Str., 1113 Sofia (mail: Sofia 1000, P.O. Box 827)/ Tel. +359 (02) 705-616 or 989-0488
Split, Croatia Cesta Mutogras 26, 21312 Podstrana (mail: P.O. Box 290, 2100)/ Tel. +385 (021) 651137
Tallinn, Estonia Luise Street 11a, 10142/ Tel. +372 6460047
Timisoara, Romania ISKCON, Porumbescu 92, 190/ Tel. +40 (056) 154776/
Vienna, Austria Bhaktivedanta-Zentrum Wien, Roetzergasse 34/3, 117/ Tel. & Fax: +43 (01) 481-9212
Vilnius, Lithuania 23-1, Raugiklos st., 2024/ Tel. +370 (2) 23-5218
Zagreb, Croatia (mail: P.O. Box 68, 10001)/ Tel. & fax: +385 (01) 3772-643

RURAL COMMUNITIES

Czech Republic Krsnuv Dvur c. 1, 25728 Chotysany/ Tel. +420 (0602) 375978
France (Bhaktivedanta Village) Chateau Bellevue, F-39700 Chatenois/ Tel. +33 (03) 8472-8235/ Fax: +33 (03) 8482-6973
France (La Nouvelle Mayapura) Domaine dÕOublaisse, 36360, Lucay le M‰le/ Tel. +33 (02) 5440-2395/ Fax: +33 (02) 5440-2893

ADDITIONAL RESTAURANTS

Aarhus, Denmark Krishnas Koekken, Mejlgade 28, 8000 Aarhus C/ Tel. +45 (08) 618-2330
Copenhagen, Denmark Govindas, N¿rre

Farimagsgade 82, DK-1364 Kbh K/ Tel. +45 3333-7444
Oslo, Norway Krishnas Cuisine, Kirkeveien 59B, 0364/ Tel. +47 (02) 260-6250
Prague, Czech Republic Govindas, Soukenicka 27, 110 00 Prague-1/ Tel. +420 (02) 2481-6631 or 2481-6016
Prague, Czech Republic Govindas, Na hrazi 5, 180 00 Prague 8-Liben/ Tel. +420 (02) 683-7226
Presov, Slovak Republic Govindas, Hlavna 70, 08001/ Tel. +0042 (191) 722 819
Radhadesh, Belgium Gopinaths Garden, Rue de Petite Somme 5, 6940 Septon-Durbuy/ Tel. +32 (086) 321421
Tallinn, Estonia Damodara, Lauteri Street 1, 10114/ Tel. +372 6442650
Vienna, Austria Govinda, Lindengasse 2A, 1070/ Tel. +43 (01) 522-2817

ASIA
INDIA
Ahmedabad, Gujarat Satellite Rd., Gandhinagar Highway Crossing, 380 054/ Tel. (079) 676-9827, 674-4944 or -4945/
Allahabad, UP Hare Krishna Dham, 161 Kashi Raj Nagar, Baluaghat 211 003/ Tel. (0532) 405294
Bangalore, KS Hare Krishna Hill, 1 ÔRÕ Block, Chord Rd., Rajaji Nagar 560 010/ Tel. (080) 332-1956/ Fax: (080) 332-4818
Bangalore, KS ISKCON Sri Jagannath Mandir, No.5 Sripuram, 1st cross, Sheshadripuram, Bangalore 560 020/ Tel. (080) 353-6867 or 226-20244 or 353-0102
Baroda, Gujarat Hare Krishna Land, Gotri Rd., 390 021/ Tel. (0265) 310630/ Fax: (0265) 331012/ E-mail: iskcon.baroda@pamho.net
Bhubaneswar, Orissa N.H. No. 5, IRC Village, 751 015/ Tel. (0674) 553517 or 555517
Bombay (see Mumbai)
Calcutta 3C Albert Rd., 700 017/ Tel. (033) 247-3757 or -6075/ Fax: (033) 247-8515
Chandigarh Hare Krishna Dham, Sector 36-B, 160 036/ Tel. (0172) 601590 or 603232/
Chennai, TN 59, Burkit Rd., T. Nagar, 600 017/ Tel. (044) 434-3266/ Fax: (044) 434-5929
Dwarka, Gujarat Bharatiya Bhavan, Devi Bhavan Rd., 361 335/ Tel. (02892) 34606/ Fax: (02892) 34319
Guwahati, Assam Ulubari Chariali, South Sarania, 781 007/ Tel. (0361) 545963
Haridwar, UP Prabhupada Ashram, G. House, Nai Basti, Bhimgoda, 249401 (mail: P.O. Box 4)/ Tel. (0133) 422655 or 425849
Hyderabad, AP Hare Krishna Land, Nampally Station Rd., 500 001/ Tel. (040) 474-4969 or -2018
Imphal, Manipur Hare Krishna Land, Airport Rd., 795 001/ Tel. (0385) 221587
Jaipur, Rajasthan ISKCON, Krishna Balaram Mandir, Dholai, Opp. Vijay Path, Mansarovar, Jaipur 302 020/ Tel. (0141) 782765
Kurukshetra, HS 369 Gudri Muhalla, Main Bazaar, 132 118/ Tel. (01744) 22806 or 23529
Lucknow, UP 1 Ashok Nagar, Guru Govind Singh Marg, 226 018
Madras (see Chennai)
Madurai, TN 37 Maninagaram Main Road, 625 001/ Tel. (0452) 746472
Mayapur, WB Shree Mayapur Chandrodaya Mandir, Shree Mayapur Dham, Dist. Nadia (mail: P.O. Box 10279, Ballyganj, Calcutta 700 019)/ Tel. (03472) 45239, 45240, or 45233/ Fax: (03472) 45238
Mumbai, Maharashtra (Bombay) Hare Krishna Land, Juhu 400 049/ Tel. (022) 620-6860/ Fax: (022) 620-5214
Mumbai, Maharashtra 7 K. M. Munshi Marg, Opposite Bharatiya Vidya Bhavan, Near Babulnath Temple, Chowpatty, 400 007/ Tel. (022) 369-7228/ Fax: (022) 367-7941
New Delhi Sant Nagar Main Rd. (Garhi), behind Nehru Place Complex (mail: P. O. Box 7061), 110 065/ Tel. (011) 623-5133/ Fax: (011) 6221-5421 or 628-0067
New Delhi 14/63, Punjabi Bagh, 110 026/ Tel. (011) 541-0782
Patna, Bihar Rajendra Nagar Rd. No. 12, 800 016/ Tel. (0612) 50765
Pune, Maharashtra 4 Tarapoor Rd., Camp, 411 001/ Tel. (0212) 667259
Puri, Orissa Bhakti Kuthi, Swargadwar/ Tel. (06752) 23740
Puri, Orissa ISKCON, Bhaktivedanta Ashram, Sipasirubuli/ Tel. (06752) 24594
Secunderabad, AP 27 St. JohnÕs Rd., 500 026/ Tel. (040) 780-5232/ Fax: (040) 814021
Silchar, Assam Ambikapatti, Silchar, Cachar Dist., 788 004
Siliguri, WB Gitalpara, 734 406/ Tel. (0353) 426619/ Fax: (0353) 526130
Sri Rangam, TN 93 Anna Mandapam Rd., A-1 Caitanya Apartments, 620 006/ Tel. (0431) 433945
Surat, Gujarat Rander Rd., Jahangirpura, 395 005/ Tel. (0261) 765891 or 765516 or 773386

Thiruvananthapuram (Trivandrum), Kerala T.C. 224/1485, WC Hospital Rd., Thycaud, 695 014/ Tel. (0471) 328197

Tirupati, AP K.T. Rd., Vinayaka Nagar, 517 507/ Tel. (08574) 20114

Udhampur, J&K Srila Prabhupada Ashram, Prabhupada Marg, Prabhupada Nagar, 182 101/ Tel. (01992) 70298

Vallabh Vidyanagar, Gujarat ISKCON, Opposite Polytechnic, 388 121/ Tel. (02692) 30796

Varanasi, UP ISKCON, B 27/80 Durgakund Rd., Near Durgakund Police Station, Varanasi 221 010/ Tel. (0542) 312062 or 222617

Vishakapatnam, AP ISKCON, 7-5-108 Pandurangapuram Beach Rd., 530 003/ Tel. (0891) 528376/ E-mail: nitaisevini@hotmail.com

Vrindavan, UP Krishna-Balaram Mandir, Bhaktivedanta Swami Marg, Raman Reti, Mathura Dist., 281 124/ Tel. (0565) 442478 or 442355/ Fax: (00565) 442596

Warangal, AP Ñ Mulugu Rd., Ayappa Pidi-pally, 506 007/ Tel. (08712) 26182

NORTH AMERICA
CANADA

Calgary, Alberta 313 Fourth Street N.E., T2E 3S3/ Tel. (403) 265-3302/ Fax: (403) 547-0795

Edmonton, Alberta 9353 35th Ave., T6E 5R5/ Tel. (403) 439-9999

Montreal, Quebec 1626 Pie IX Boulevard, H1V 2C5/ Tel. & fax: (514) 521-1301

Ottawa, Ontario 212 Somerset St. E., K1N 6V4/ Tel. (613) 565-6544/ Fax: (613) 565-2575

Regina, Saskatchewan 1279 Retallack St., S4T 2H8/ Tel. (306) 525-1640

Toronto, Ontario 243 Avenue Rd., M5R 2J6/ Tel. (416) 922-5415/ Fax: (416) 922-1021

Vancouver, B.C. 5462 S.E. Marine Dr., Burnaby V5J 3G8/ Tel. (604) 433-9728/ Fax: (604) 431-7251

Govindas Restaurant: Tel. (604) 433-2428/ Fax: (604) 431-7251

RURAL COMMUNITY

Ashcroft, B.C. Saranagati Dhama (mail: P.O. Box 99, V0K 1A0, attn: Uttama Devi Dasi)/ Tel. (250) 453-2397/ Fax: (250) 453-2622 [attn: (250) 453-2397]

U.S.A.

Atlanta, Georgia 1287 South Ponce de Leon Ave. N.E., 30306/ Tel. (404) 378-9234/ Fax: (404) 373-3381

Austin, Texas 10700 Jonwood Way, 78753/ Tel. (512) 835-2121

Baltimore, Maryland 200 Bloomsbury Ave., Catonsville, 21228/ Tel. (410) 744-4069 or 719-6738/ Tel. & fax: (410) 744-1624

Berkeley, California 2334 Stuart Street, 94705/ Tel. (510) 540-9215

Boise, Idaho 1615 Martha St., 83706/ Tel. (208) 344-4274

Boston, Massachusetts 72 Commonwealth Ave., 02116/ Tel. (617) 247-8611/ Fax: (617) 266-3744

Charlotte, North Carolina 9408-D Lexington Circle, 28213/ Tel. (704)549-4603

Chicago, Illinois 1716 W. Lunt Ave., 60626/ Tel. (773) 973-0900/ Fax: (773) 973-0526

Columbus, Ohio 379 W. Eighth Ave., 43201/ Tel. (614) 421-1661/ Fax: (614) 294-0545

Dallas, Texas 5430 Gurley Ave., 75223/ Tel. (214) 827-6330/ Fax: (214) 823-7264

Denver, Colorado 1400 Cherry St., 80220/ Tel. (303) 333-5461/ Fax: (303) 321-9052

Detroit, Michigan 383 Lenox Ave., 48215/ Tel. (313) 824-6000/ Fax: (313) 822-3748

Gainesville, Florida 214 N.W. 14th St., 32603/ Tel. (352) 336-4183/ Fax: (352) 379-2923

Hartford, Connecticut 1683 Main St., E. Hartford, 06108/ Tel. & fax: (860) 289-7252

Honolulu, Hawaii 51 Coelho Way, 96817/ Tel. (808) 595-3947/ Fax: (808) 595-3433

Houston, Texas 1320 W. 34th St., 77018/ Tel. (713) 686-4482/ Fax: (713) 686-0669

Kansas City, Missouri Rupanuga Vedic College (Mens Seminary), 5201 The Paseo, 64110/ Tel. (816) 361-6167 or (800) 340-5286/ Fax: (816) 361-0509

Laguna Beach, California 285 Legion St., 92651/ Tel. (949) 494-7029

Long Island, New York 197 S. Ocean Avenue, Freeport, 11520/ Tel. (516) 223-4909

Los Angeles, California 3764 Watseka Ave., 90034/ Tel. (310) 836-2676/ Fax: (310) 839-2715

Los Angeles, California 3520-3526 Slauson Ave., 90043/ Tel. (323) 295-1517

Miami, Florida 3220 Virginia St., 33133 (mail: P.O. Box 337, Coconut Grove, FL 33233)/ Tel. (305) 442-7218/ Fax: (305) 444-7145

New Orleans, Louisiana 2936 Esplanade Ave., 70119/ Tel. (504) 486-3583

New York, New York 305 Schermerhorn St., Brooklyn, 11217/ Tel. (718) 855-6714/ Fax: (718) 875-6127

New York, New York 26 Second Avenue, 10003 (mail: P. O. Box 2509, New York, NY 10009/ Tel. (212) 420-1130
New York, New York 114-37 Lefferts Blvd., Queens 11420 / Tel. & fax: (718) 848-9010
Philadelphia, Pennsylvania 41 West Allens Lane, 19119/ Tel. (215) 247-4600/ Fax: (215) 247-8702
Philadelphia, Pennsylvania 1408 South St., 19148/ Tel. (215) 985-9335
Phoenix, Arizona 100 S. Weber Dr., Chandler, 85226/ Tel. (480) 705-4900/ Fax: (602) 705-4901
Portland, Oregon 2353 SE 54th Ave., Portland, OR 97215/ Tel. (503) 236-0417
Queens, New York 114-37 Lefferts Blvd., 11420 / Tel. & fax: (718) 848-9010
St. Louis, Missouri 3926 Lindell Blvd., 63108/ Tel. (314) 535-8085/ Fax: (314) 535-0672
San Diego, California 1030 Grand Ave., Pacific Beach, 92109/ Tel. (858) 483-2500/ Fax: (858) 483-0941
San Jose, California 2990 Union Ave., 95124/ Tel. (408) 559-3197
Seattle, Washington 1420 228th Ave. S.E., Issaquah, 98027/ Tel. (425) 391-3293/ Fax: (425) 868-8928
Spanish Fork, Utah Krishna Temple Project & KHQN Radio, 8628 S. State Rd., 84660/ Tel. (801) 798-3559/ Fax: (801) 798-9121
Tallahassee, Florida 1323 Nylic St., 32304/ Tel. & fax: (850) 224-3803
Tampa, Florida 1205 E. Giddens Ave., 33603/ Tel. (813) 234-8841
Towaco, New Jersey 100 Jacksonville Rd. (mail: P.O. Box 109), 07082/ Tel. & fax: (973) 299-0970
Tucson, Arizona 711 E. Blackledge Dr., 85719/ Tel. (520) 792-0630/ Fax: (520) 791-0906
Washington, D.C. 1009 Noyes Dr., Silver Spring, MD 20910/ Tel. (301) 562-9662 or 765-8155/ Fax: (301) 765-8157
Washington, D.C. 10310 Oaklyn Dr., Potomac, Maryland 20854/ Tel. (301) 299-2100/ Fax: (301) 299-5025

AUSTRALASIA
AUSTRALIA
Adelaide 25 Le Hunte St., Kilburn, SA 5084/ Tel. +61 (08) 8359-5120/ Fax: (08) 8359-5149
Brisbane 95 Bank Rd., Graceville (mail: P.O. Box 83, Indooroopilly), QLD 4068/ Tel. +61 (07) 3379-5455/ Fax: +61 (07) 3379-5880
Canberra 1 Quick St., Ainslie, ACT 2602 (mail: P.O. Box 1411, Canberra, ACT 2601)/ Tel. & fax: +61 (02) 6262-6208/
Melbourne 197 Danks St. (mail: P.O. Box 125), Albert Park , VIC 3206/ Tel. +61 (03) 9699-5122/ Fax: +61 (03) 9690-4093
Newcastle 28 Bull St., Mayfield NSW 2304/ Tel. +61 (02) 4967-7000
Perth 144 Railway Parade (corner of The Strand) [mail: P.O. Box 102], Bayswater, WA 6053/ Tel. +61 (08) 9370-1552 Fax: +61 (08) 9272-6636
Sydney 180 Falcon St., North Sydney, NSW 2060 (mail: P.O. Box 459, Cammeray, NSW 2062)/Tel. +61 (02) 9959-4558/ Fax:+61(02) 9957-1893

RURAL COMMUNITIES
Bambra (New Nandagram) Oak Hill, Deans Marsh Road, VIC 3241/ Tel +61 (03) 5288-7383
Cessnock, New Gokula Farm, Lewis Lane (off Mount View Rd., Millfield [mail: P.O. Box 399, Cessnock), NSW 2325/ Tel. +61 (02) 4998-1800/ Fax: (Sydney temple)
Murwillumbah (New Govardhana) Tyalgum Rd., Eungella (mail: P.O. Box 685),Murwillumbah NSW 2484/ Tel. & fax: +61 (02) 6672-6579/

RESTAURANTS
Adelaide Hare Krishna Food for Life, 79 Hindley St., SA 5000/ Tel. +61 (08) 8231-5258
Brisbane Govindas, 99 Elizabeth St., 1st floor, QLD 4000/ Tel. +61 (07) 3210-0255
Brisbane Hare Krishna Food for Life, 190 Brunswick St., Fortitude Valley, QLD/ Tel. +61 (07) 3854-1016
Darlinghurst Govindas Upstairs,112 Darlinghurst Road, NSW 2010/ Tel. +61 (02) 9380-5162
Melbourne Crossways, 1st Floor, 123 Swanston St., VIC 3000/ Tel. +61 (03) 9650-2939
Melbourne Gopals, 139 Swanston St., VIC 3000/ Tel. +61 (03) 9650-1578
New Castle Krishnas Vegetarian Cafe, 110 King Street, corner of King & Wolf Streets, NSW 2300 Tel. +61 (02) 4929-6900
Perth Hare Krishna Food for Life, 200 William St., Northbridge, WA 6003/ Tel. +61 (08) 9227-1684

NEW ZEALAND, FIJI AND PAPUA NEW GUINEA
Christchurch, NZ 83 Bealey Ave. (mail: P.O.

Box 25-190)/ Tel. +64 (03) 366-5174/ Fax: +64 (03) 366-1965
Labasa, Fiji Delailabasa (mail: P.O. Box 133)/ Tel. +679 812912
Lautoka, Fiji 5 Tavewa Ave. (mail: P.O. Box 125)/ Tel. +679 664112/ Fax: +679 663039
Port Moresby, Papua New Guinea Section 23, Lot 46, Gordonia St., Hohola (mail: P.O. Box 571, POM NCD)/ Tel. +675 259213
Rakiraki, Fiji Rewasa (mail: P.O. Box 204)/ Tel. +679 694243
Suva, Fiji Joyce Place, Off Pilling Rd., Nasinu 71 2 miles (mail: P.O. Box 2183, Govt. Bldgs.)/ Tel. +679 393 599
Wellington, NZ 105 Newlands Rd., Newlands (mail: P.O. Box 2753)/ Tel. +64 (04) 478-1414

RURAL COMMUNITY
Auckland, NZ (New Varshan) Hwy. 28, Riverhead, next to Huapai Golf Course (mail: R.D. 2, Kumeu)/ Tel. +64 (09) 412-8075/ Fax: +64 (09) 412-7130

RESTAURANTS
Auckland, NZ GopalÕs, 246 Queen St./ Tel. +64 (09) 306-4143
Labasa, Fiji Hare Krishna Restaurant, Naseakula Road/ Tel. +679 811364
Lautoka, Fiji GopalÕs, Corner of Yasawa St. and Naviti St./ Tel. +679 662990
Suva, Fiji Hare Krishna Vegetarian Restaurant, Dolphins FNPF Place, Victoria Parade/ Tel. +679 314154/ E-mail: vdas@govnet.gov.fj
Suva, Fiji Hare Krishna Vegetarian Restaurant, Opposite University of the South Pacific, Laucala Bay Rd./ Tel. +679 311683

COMMONWEALTH OF INDEPENDENT STATES
RUSSIA
Ekaterinburg 620078, G. Ekaterinburg, per. Otdelnij 5DK VOG/ Tel. +7 (3432) 74-2200 or 49-5262
Irkutsk st. Krimskaya 6A/ Tel. (3952) 38-71-32 or 3240-62
Kazan 13, Sortirovochnaya st, pos.Yudino/ Tel. +7 (8432) 55-2529 or 42-9991
Krasnodar 418, Stepnaya st., selo Elizavetinskoye, Krsnodarski krai/ Tel. +7 (8612) 50-1694
Kurjinovo 8, Shosseinaya st., pos. Ershovo, Urupski region, Karachayevo-Cherkessia
Moscow 8/3, Khoroshevskoye sh. (mail: P.O. Box 69), 125284/ Tel. +7 (095) 255-6711/ Tel. & fax: +7 (095) 9453317
Moscow Nekrasovsky pos., Dmitrovsky reg., 141700/ Tel. +7 (095) 577-8543, -8601, or -8775/ Fax: +7 (095) 4464746
Murmansk 16, Frolova st. (mail: P.O. Box 5823)/ Tel. +7 (8152) 58-9284
Nijny Novgorod 14b, Chernigovskaya st./ Tel. +7 (8312) 30-5197 or 25-2592
Novorossiysk 117, Shillerovskaya st./ Tel. +7 (86134) 38-926 or 51-415
Novosibirsk 18/2 Kholodilynaya st., 630001/ Tel. +7 (3832) 46-2655 or -2666
Omsk 664099, 42 10th Severnaya st. (mail: P.O. Box 8741)/ Tel. +7 (3812) 24-5310 or 41-4051
Perm 12, Verhnekuryinskaya st., 614065/ Tel. +7 (3422) 33-5740 or 27-0681
Rostov-na-Donu 84/1, Saryana st., 344025 (mail: P.O. Box 64, 344007)/ Tel. & fax: +7 (8632) 51-0456
Samara 122, Aeroportovskoye sh., Zubchininovka/ Tel. +7 (8462) 97-0318 or -0323
Simbirsk 10, Glinki st., 432002/ Tel. +7 (8422) 21-4016
Sochi Vinogradnaya 108
Ulan-Ude 670013, Prirechnaya str. 23/ Tel. +7 (3012) 30-795
Vladimir 60000, Nikolo-Galeyskaya st. 56/25/ Tel. +7 (0922) 32-6726

RESTAURANTS
Ekaterinburg Sankirtana, 33 Bardina st./ Tel. +7 (3432) 41-2737
St. Petersburg GovindaÕs, 58, Angliysky pr., 190008/ Tel. +7 (812) 113-7896
Vladivostok GopalÕs, 10/12, Oleansky pr./ Tel. +7 (4232) 26-8943

UKRAINE
Dnepropetrovsk Kalininskiy spusk 39/ Tel. +73 (0562) 42-3631 or 45-4709
Donetsk 22, Rubensa st., Makeyevka 339018/ Tel. +380 (0622) 94-9104 or -3140
Kharkov 43, Verhnegiyovskaya st., Holodnaya Gora, 310015/ Tel. +380 (0572) 20-2167 or 72-6869
Kiev Dmitrievskaya, 21-13/ Tel. +380 (044) 219-1041 or -1042/ Tel. & fax: +380 (044) 244-4934
Kiev 16, Zorany per., 254078/ Tel. +380 (044) 433-8312, or 434-7028 or -5533
Nikolaev 5-8, Sudostroitelny per., 327052/ Tel. +380 (0510) 35-1734
Vinnica 5, Chkalov st., 28601/ Tel. +380 (0432) 32-3152